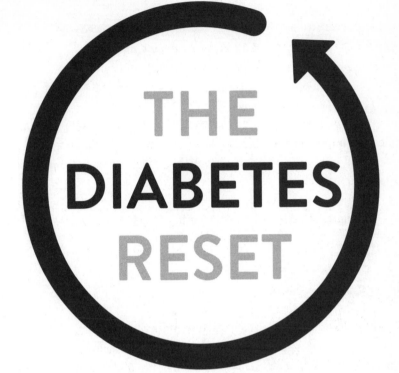

THE DIABETES RESET

Avoid It. Control It.
Even Reverse It.

A Doctor's Scientific Program

GEORGE L. KING, M.D.

WITH ROYCE FLIPPIN

WORKMAN PUBLISHING · NEW YORK

Library of Congress Cataloging-in-Publication Data is available.

ISBN 978-0-7611-7592-6

Design by Jean-Marc Troadec

Workman books are available at special discounts when purchased in bulk
for premiums and sales promotions as well as for fund-raising or educational
use. Special editions or book excerpts also can be created to specification.
For details, contact the Special Sales Director at the address below, or send
an email to specialmarkets@workman.com.

Workman Publishing Company, Inc.
225 Varick Street
New York, NY 10014-4381
workman.com

Printed in the United States of America

First printing December 2014

10 9 8 7 6 5 4 3 2 1

I dedicate this book to my wife, Diana, and my sons, Benjamin and Adam, for their lifetime of support. I also want to express my appreciation to all the investigators, health providers, and patients with diabetes at JOSLIN DIABETES CENTER and everywhere for their passion and hard work in managing this disease.

CONTENTS

ACKNOWLEDGMENTS

I would like to thank my literary agent, Katherine Cowles, who had the original vision for this book, and without whom *The Diabetes Reset* would not have been written. I also want to thank my assistants, Daad Abraham and Karen Lau, for their extensive efforts in the research and writing of this book. In addition, I am grateful to the Joslin researchers and clinicians who generously shared their time and expertise, and to the administrators at Joslin for their support of this project. Finally, I offer my special thanks to Royce Flippin, my collaborator on this project, and to the editors and production team at Workman Publishing, especially Mary Ellen O'Neill, for their fine work in bringing this book to publication.

(Note: Dr. King will be donating 50% of his proceeds from *The Diabetes Reset* to the Joslin Medalist Study and Joslin's Asian American Diabetes Institute.)

INTRODUCTION:
THE DIABETES RESET PROMISE

I f you're reading this book, it's very likely that you or someone close to you is struggling with blood glucose levels. It could be that your fasting blood glucose level was higher than it should have been at your last checkup—perhaps in the prediabetes range of 100 to 125 mg/dL (milligrams per deciliter), indicating you have impaired glucose tolerance and are at high risk of developing diabetes. Your fasting blood glucose may even be more than 125 mg/dL, which is considered the threshold for type 2 diabetes.

You may also have gotten test results showing that your hemoglobin A1C levels, which measure your average blood glucose over the past several months, are elevated—meaning they were either between 5.7% and 6.4%, the range for prediabetes, or 6.5% or higher, signaling that you may actually have diabetes.

Learning that your blood glucose levels are too high can be bewildering, even frightening. Because both type 2 diabetes and its precursor, prediabetes, tend to develop slowly over many years, it's tempting to think that once you've been diagnosed with one of these conditions, there's not much you can do except take diabetes medication and hope for the best. As a lifelong diabetes researcher, however, I want to assure you that *nothing could be further from the truth*. In reality, you can *always* take steps to improve your body's response to insulin and "reset" your ability to metabolize the glucose in your blood—starting today.

This simple statement has profound implications. It means that if you have prediabetes, not only can you prevent your condition from progressing to diabetes, but in many cases you can actually reverse course and bring your glucose metabolism back to normal. Even if you've already been diagnosed with type 2 diabetes, you can still significantly improve your body's natural glucose metabolism and dramatically reduce—and in some cases even eliminate—your need for metformin, synthetic insulin, or other diabetes drugs.

The promise of *The Diabetes Reset* is equally simple: If you follow the evidence-based approaches in this book, you will begin seeing immediate improvements in your body's ability to metabolize blood glucose—improvements that will continue to grow over time. At the same time, you will also see remarkable improvements in your overall health. In addition to becoming lighter and fitter, you will find yourself eating the types of foods that human beings have thrived on for thousands of years. You'll also sleep better at night, experience less stress during the day, and have a more balanced immune system that fights off illness without overreacting. And because impaired blood glucose control is a major risk factor for cardiovascular disease, you will be taking a major step toward improved heart health as well.

Glucose and the Goldilocks Principle

There are only 4 grams of glucose—just enough to fill a teaspoon—circulating at any given time in the bloodstream of an average-weight person. But keeping that small amount of glucose constant is vitally important to your health. When it comes to your blood glucose level, the Goldilocks principle holds—you want it to be in the "just right" range, no lower than 70 mg/dL and no higher than 100 mg/dL when you wake up in the morning, and no higher than 140 gm/dL one to two hours after eating a meal. Normally, your body is programmed to keep glucose safely

The Diabetes Reset: Not for Type 2 Diabetes Only!

Although the diabetes-control strategies in *The Diabetes Reset* have been written primarily for people with prediabetes or type 2 diabetes, they will also benefit people with type 1 diabetes and pregnant women who may be at risk of gestational diabetes. By using these approaches to increase insulin sensitivity, type 1 diabetics can enhance their glucose control and also reduce the amount of insulin medication they require, which in turn will make it easier to control their weight. At the same time, the recommendations contained in this book will enhance their overall health and reduce risk of vascular complications. Similarly, pregnant women can use these approaches to reduce the risk of developing gestational diabetes.

within this range. When glucose levels rise, the body automatically produces more insulin to speed the absorption of this glucose into the body's tissues. When glucose levels dip toward the lower end of this range, the liver releases stored glucose into the bloodstream, while the pancreas stops producing insulin and may instead secrete glucagon, a hormone that induces the liver to manufacture still more glucose.

If this system falters and you become *hyperglycemic,* meaning that your blood glucose levels are consistently elevated, this excess glucose will begin attacking your nerve endings and the walls of your blood vessels. Over time, this can lead to neurological problems, damage to the eyes, kidneys, inner ear, and other organs, and increased risk of heart attack and stroke. Although these complications are typically associated with diabetes—defined as a fasting blood glucose of 126 mg/dL or higher or a postmeal glucose level of 200 mg/dL or above—people with prediabetes (a 100 mg/dL to 125 mg/dL fasting glucose level, or 140 mg/dL to 200 mg/dL following a meal) can also be at increased risk for these conditions.

If blood glucose levels fall too low, on the other hand, a condition known as *hypoglycemia,* your health can also suffer. Because the brain relies completely on blood glucose for fuel, and requires a lot of it (when you're in a sedentary fasting state, your brain consumes a whopping 60% of your total blood glucose supply), it is quickly affected by low glucose levels. People typically begin noticing the mental effects of low blood sugar as their glucose levels drop below 70 mg/dL. These may include feelings of irritability, anxiety, and difficulty concentrating. Low blood sugar can also cause headaches, fatigue, blurred vision, sweating, an elevated heartbeat, tremors, and hunger pangs. If glucose levels drop further still, it can lead to fainting, seizures, coma, and even death. People who take insulin medication for type 1 or type 2 diabetes are at particular risk for low blood glucose because injected insulin can push glucose levels too low if it's administered at the wrong time or in the wrong dose.

If you notice signs of low blood glucose, you should immediately ingest 15 grams of fast-acting carbohydrate, such as: 4 ounces of fruit juice, 6 ounces of regular soda, three to four glucose tablets, one small box of raisins, 1 tablespoon of honey or syrup, or seven gummy bears.

Why Is My Blood Glucose Too High?

W hen your blood glucose levels start to rise, it's an indication that several related things are occurring inside your body. First, your body's insulin—the hormone that has primary responsibility for keeping your blood glucose within a normal range—is no longer working as effectively as it should because specific tissues aren't fully responding to its actions. This reduction in *insulin sensitivity,* commonly referred to as *insulin resistance,* has different effects depending on where it occurs.

- In your muscles, where most blood glucose is burned or stored, insulin resistance makes it harder for glucose to enter the muscle cells. The result is that more insulin is needed to help the muscles absorb glucose. If not enough insulin is available, then excess glucose is left circulating in your bloodstream while less glucose passes into your muscles to help power them. For most people, insulin resistance in the muscles is what starts them on the path to type 2 diabetes.

- In your liver, which both stores and manufactures glucose, insulin acts to suppress glucose production. When the liver becomes insulin resistant, however, insulin's suppressive effect on glucose production is reduced, causing excess glucose to be released from the liver into the bloodstream.

- The third major "target" of insulin is the body's fat tissues. Insulin works on the fat cells to suppress the breakdown of fat stores into fatty acids for use as fuel. When fat tissue becomes insulin resistant, this suppressive effect is reduced, inhibiting the fat storage process—which, as we'll see shortly, can lead to even more insulin resistance by contributing to fat buildup in the muscles and liver.

Although insulin resistance works differently in the muscles, fat, and liver, the result is the same: The body must pump out greater amounts of insulin on an ongoing basis in an attempt to keep blood glucose levels under control. Insulin resistance can exist for many years without causing a noticeable rise in blood glucose levels (although even then it places the insulin-resistant individual at increased risk for cardiovascular disease). In a sizable percentage of people with insulin resistance, however, there comes a time when the beta cells in their pancreas—the cells that manufacture insulin—can no longer make enough insulin to overcome their decreased insulin sensitivity.

When this occurs, your blood glucose levels become elevated and you cross the threshold to prediabetes. If your pancreas continues to fall behind, the next step will be type 2 diabetes. With your body unable to manufacture enough insulin to metabolize all the glucose in your blood, your blood glucose will remain at unhealthy levels unless you begin taking diabetes medication or start pursuing some serious antidiabetes lifestyle strategies—such as the ones outlined in this book.

Unraveling the Causes of Type 2 Diabetes

At the most basic level, then, type 2 diabetes is a simple two-step process: First, you develop insulin resistance, requiring more insulin to be produced to keep glucose levels under control. Second, your insulin production begins to fall short, causing glucose levels to rise. This sounds straightforward enough. But exactly *why* this two-step process occurs in some people and not others has remained a medical mystery until fairly recently. We knew, for example, that being overweight contributes significantly to type 2 diabetes risk (as evidenced by the fact that 80% of people with type 2 diabetes are overweight or obese) and that getting regular exercise appears to improve glucose control and lessen type 2 diabetes risk, but the mechanisms behind these connections weren't clear.

That situation has altered dramatically over the past twenty years. Thanks to major advances in our ability to understand and investigate the complex biochemical reactions that regulate our bodies, we are starting to gain a fairly good understanding of the causes of insulin resistance—which, it turns out, is a complex, multifaceted phenomenon. We're beginning to unravel some of the causes of pancreatic failure as well, which offers promise not only for the prevention and treatment of prediabetes and type 2 diabetes, but also for the treatment of people with type 1 diabetes—an autoimmune disorder that typically strikes early in life, attacking the insulin-producing cells in the pancreas to the point where it can manufacture little or no insulin at all.

In *The Diabetes Reset,* I've drawn on these latest findings to provide eight evidence-based strategies for reversing the insulin resistance process and preserving the insulin-producing function of your pancreas. In these eight strategy chapters, I'll describe in detail many of the exciting discoveries being made by diabetes researchers about the importance of diet, weight loss, exercise, stress, and other key factors. First, though, I want to share our current knowledge about the underlying causes of prediabetes and type 2 diabetes.

The Four Drivers of Insulin Resistance

Much of the discussion around diabetes centers on carbohydrates— the nutrient that your body converts into glucose. And it's certainly true that persistently high levels of glucose in the bloodstream are what actually cause many of the physical problems associated with diabetes by damaging the nerves and the blood vessels that feed the heart, kidneys, eyes, and other vital organs. But elevated blood lipids in the form of total cholesterol and LDL cholesterol (which are linked mainly to dietary consumption of fat rather than carbohydrates) are also important risk factors in diabetic patients. What's more, we now know that elevated blood glucose levels and blood lipids are actually driven by insulin resistance, caused in varying degrees by the following factors:

- Fat accumulation in muscle and liver tissue
- Mitochondrial dysfunction due to oxidative stress
- Systemic and local inflammation
- Psychological stress

All of these factors interfere with the biological action of insulin in various ways. Here is a quick look at their insulin-blunting effects:

FAT ACCUMULATION IN MUSCLE AND LIVER TISSUE

The accumulation of droplets of fat in the muscles and liver—known as ectopic fat—is now understood to be an important cause of insulin resistance and, ultimately, type 2 diabetes. For many people, this accumulation of fat inside the muscles may well represent the very first step on the path toward prediabetes and type 2 diabetes. When lipids collect in the muscle cells, they interfere with the insulin-signaling process that enables glucose to be transported into those cells.

Exactly which fat-related compounds are responsible for short-circuiting insulin's actions is still being investigated, but the overall link is clear. In fact, if you were to measure the amount of fat accumulation inside someone's muscle cells, that would give you a better idea of how insulin resistant he or she is than many other commonly used measures of diabetes risk, including body mass index and waist circumference.

In general, liver insulin resistance is thought to occur at a later stage than muscle insulin resistance in the progression toward type 2 diabetes, but fat deposits also appear to play an important role here. A number of studies have shown a close association between fat buildup in the liver—known as nonalcoholic fatty liver disease—and increased insulin resistance in the liver.

How do these excess fats get into the muscles and liver? One chief source appears to be obesity. As a person gets steadily fatter, his or her body becomes less able to store all the excess energy in its main deposits of fat tissues, and the fat cells themselves become more prone to metabolizing into free fatty acids. These fatty acids then circulate through the bloodstream, where they are available to be taken up by other organs. This is particularly true of abdominal fat, which appears to release the lion's share of fatty acids into the bloodstream. The fatty acid effect is heightened by a vicious cycle that develops as the fat cells become insulin resistant as well. When less glucose is able to enter these cells, this further suppresses the fat-storing effects of insulin and promotes the additional breakdown of fat tissue into fatty acids, adding to the amount of available fatty acids in the blood.

A high-fat diet—including even a single high-fat meal—can also increase blood levels of fatty acids if the amount of fat consumed exceeds the body's ability to store it away as fat tissue, resulting in almost immediate increases in insulin resistance. In research projects in which human subjects were given infusions of fat designed to raise the levels of fatty acids in their bloodstream, their muscles' ability to respond to insulin and utilize glucose dropped measurably within just a few hours. Likewise, animal studies have found that eating a high-fat diet quickly leads to increased fat levels and insulin resistance inside the liver. Obesity seems to contribute to this phenomenon by impairing the body's ability to store dietary fat as fat tissue.

Fat buildup in the muscles can also occur when the muscles' ability to metabolize, or oxidize, fatty acids for fuel is impaired, causing fats to accumulate inside the muscle cells. Normal-weight people with a strong family history of type 2 diabetes have been found to have insulin resistance related to this sort of muscle impairment, probably for genetic reasons. The muscles' ability to oxidize fat can also decline with age, and similar muscle impairments have been found in elderly individuals who are insulin resistant despite being normal weight. Physical inactivity can also reduce your muscles' ability to metabolize fat.

The first three strategy chapters of *The Diabetes Reset* take direct aim at this source of insulin resistance. Eating a low-fat, high-fiber diet—the strategy outlined in Strategy Chapter 1—minimizes the amount of fatty acids in the bloodstream and, through delaying absorption of fat and other digested food plus metabolites of gut flora in the colon, may actually change the nature of the fats in peripheral tissues. Strategy Chapter 2 directly targets weight loss, which reduces overall body fat stores—a major source of ectopic fat—and has also been shown to directly improve liver insulin resistance. Strategy Chapter 3 focuses on exercise, which has been shown to sharply enhance the ability of the muscles to metabolize fatty acids, leading to a reduction of fat content in the muscle cells and a dramatic increase in muscle insulin sensitivity.

MITOCHONDRIAL DYSFUNCTION DUE TO OXIDATIVE STRESS

Mitochondria are the microscopic "batteries" that fuel all of your cells, which in turn are the building blocks of the body. This means that mitochondria, in essence, are your body's power supply. Glucose and fat are the fuels used to generate energy in the mitochondria. During this energy generation process, molecules known as reactive oxygen species (ROS), which include "free radicals" and other types of highly reactive oxygen molecules, are produced. Under normal circumstances, these ROS are promptly neutralized by the body's natural antioxidant mechanisms.

When there is excessive fat or glucose in the cells, however, or when other deficiencies occur in the antioxidative process, excessive ROS can be produced, resulting in what is known as oxidative stress. This stress can cause mitochondrial dysfunction, which in turn can cause the cells to become insulin resistant.

The general idea that people can be harmed by mitochondrial dysfunction due to oxidative stress has been around for quite a while. The popularity of antioxidant supplements, which are taken to neutralize ROS, is based partly on this idea. ROS are charged oxygen particles, or ions, that interact very readily with surrounding atoms. The activities of ROS aren't all bad—in fact, many ROS interactions are essential for good health—but the oxidative stress that occurs when excessive amounts of ROS interact with nearby tissue can cause serious damage on the cellular level. Among other things, oxidative stress is thought to be central to the aging process and many degenerative diseases.

The interest around oxidative stress and diabetes has emerged from findings that these charged particles can interfere with the insulin-signaling process and can also damage the beta cells of the pancreas. Some of the ways they seem to do this are related to the other two drivers of insulin resistance, excessive fat buildup and inflammation. One source of ROS is the combination of overeating and lack of exercise, which places stress on the mitochondria. When we take in more energy than we expend, the buildup of fats and glucose inside muscle and fat cells cause ROS to form in these cells. In fact, it's been suggested that insulin resistance may actually be the body's attempt to defend against this ROS overactivity by slowing down the mitochondrial actions in these tissues.

In Strategy Chapter 8, I'll offer some ideas about how you can take advantage of these findings—and help increase your insulin sensitivity—by stimulating production of your body's many natural antioxidants. I'll also explain why this approach, which neutralizes oxidative stress on the cellular level, works far better than taking supplements of a single antioxidant such as Vitamin E.

SYSTEMIC AND LOCAL INFLAMMATION

One of the most remarkable diabetes-related discoveries in recent years has been the role that inflammation appears to play in promoting insulin resistance. We now know that body fat, far from being an inert storage bank for energy, as was once thought, is a chemical factory, producing fifty or more types of molecules that help trigger other biological processes in the body. As you start to gain excess weight and your fat cells begin to grow in size, this mix of molecules begins to change and your body fat begins to pump out a greater amount of pro-inflammatory chemicals called cytokines. At the same time, these supersized fat cells attract immune system cells called macrophages, which also secrete cytokines. This combined effect is powerful enough, in fact, that when someone becomes obese, his or her body can shift to a state of chronic, low-level inflammation.

Scientists have also found that many of these cytokines appear to contribute directly to insulin resistance by interfering with the insulin-signaling process on the cellular level, contributing directly to insulin resistance in the body's organs. Others stimulate additional inflammatory processes, which have their own impact on insulin resistance. These cytokines also travel through the bloodstream, causing chronic systemic inflammation (a low-level inflammatory response throughout the body that also contributes to insulin resistance and can damage the pancreas as well). Systemic inflammation can also cause localized inflammation in the muscles and the liver—both of which may contribute to insulin resistance in these organs. In addition, the inflammatory effect on the liver creates a vicious cycle because liver inflammation causes more fat to accumulate in the liver, making it more insulin resistant still.

Although obesity-related inflammation appears to play a significant role in insulin resistance and the development of type 2 diabetes, other factors can contribute to the production of inflammatory cytokines as well—particularly a high-fat diet, which can trigger the release of cytokines in the bloodstream and can also encourage the absorption of certain inflammatory toxins from the intestinal tract. Other chronic inflammatory states have been linked to increased risk of type 2 diabetes, including periodontal disease, kidney disease, lack of sleep, and certain autoimmune conditions such as psoriasis, rheumatoid arthritis, and asthma. Gestational diabetes, which is triggered by hormones produced during pregnancy, also appears related to inflammatory processes to some degree. In addition, a great deal of excitement has been generated recently around the findings that gut bacteria can affect body weight, possibly by increasing inflammation in the gut. Finally, inflammation caused by elevated glucose levels and by excess body fat has been directly implicated in the impairment of beta cell function in the pancreas.

Again, the strategies I present in *The Diabetes Reset* are designed to attack the issue of inflammation-related insulin resistance head-on. Although my chapters on weight loss and eating a low-fat diet can clearly help reduce the threat of inflammation from obesity and dietary fat, I've also devoted the entirety of Strategy Chapter 5 to explaining the link between inflammation and diabetes in detail, as well as providing a wealth of other inflammation-fighting tips. Strategy Chapters 6 and 7, which address the importance of getting enough good-quality sleep and managing psychological stress, are also related to inflammation, in large part because both lack of sleep and chronic stress are associated with increased inflammatory activity.

PSYCHOLOGICAL STRESS

Both the behavioral and chemical impact of chronic stress and the mood disorders it is linked to, depression and anxiety, can contribute to insulin resistance, pancreas malfunction, and the progression of type 2 diabetes. In Strategy Chapter 7, I go into detail about how chronic stress affects your glucose metabolism negatively—due in large part to the effects of the stress hormone cortisol—and steps you can take to counter it.

Preserving Your Beta Cells

As I noted earlier, insulin resistance is the impairment of the glucose disposal process. In order for insulin resistance to progress to prediabetes or type 2 diabetes, however, the beta cells of the pancreas also must become defective to the point where they can no longer produce enough insulin to cope with the increased levels of glucose in your bloodstream. Why this happens to some people and not others is still not clear. Scientists believe that genetics probably plays a significant role—some people are born with fewer beta cells or beta cells that function less well or are more susceptible to stress. At the same time, beta cells can also be damaged by the very same things that cause insulin resistance: excess fats in your system, inflammation, and oxidative stress. This means that the strategies outlined in *The Diabetes Reset* will help preserve your beta cells as well, both by directly protecting your pancreas from these various stresses and by reducing insulin resistance—which puts less pressure on the pancreas to produce insulin and also helps prevent elevated glucose levels, which are yet another source of beta cell damage.

The Diabetes Reset: Repositioning Yourself on the Diabetes Pathway

No two cases of type 2 diabetes (or prediabetes) are exactly alike. The fact that so many different factors contribute to insulin resistance and beta cell dysfunction means that your own glucose control problems are caused by a unique combination of these factors. The reason for this is that no two people's physiologies are identical: Some people can put on excess body fat without triggering the same level of inflammation as others. Some people's muscle cells burn fat more efficiently than others, minimizing the accumulation of fat inside those cells. Some have higher natural levels of antioxidants, while others produce more stress hormones when they're in an anxiety-provoking situation. This is why *The Diabetes Reset* provides a wide range of diabetes-fighting strategies.

In Part Two of this book, I'll provide a framework for implementing these various strategies and monitoring your progress. As I mentioned earlier, type 2 diabetes typically develops over many years. During that time, a person passes through various stages of metabolic dysfunction—a continuum I think of as the "diabetes pathway." Movement along this pathway also varies from person to person: When a person develops insulin resistance, it can take years for this condition to progress to prediabetes, and years more until their insulin shortfall reaches the point where they are diagnosed with type 2 diabetes. What's more, some people with insulin resistance never get prediabetes, and some people with prediabetes manage to avoid developing type 2 diabetes. In some cases, this is due to the fact their genetic vulnerability is limited. In other cases, they are able to halt—and even reverse—their movement down that path by employing the strategies presented in *The Diabetes Reset*.

The important thing to realize is that it's never too soon to begin taking steps to improve your insulin sensitivity and protect your pancreatic function. The earlier on the diabetes pathway you are, the easier it is to stop your forward progress and start reversing direction. That's why I strongly recommend the strategies in this book for *anyone* who thinks he may be at risk for type 2 diabetes, either because he has early signs of impaired glucose tolerance or because he has significant risk factors such as obesity or a family history of type 2 diabetes—particularly a parent or sibling with the condition.

On the other hand, no matter *how far* you've progressed along the diabetes pathway, you can still improve your health and begin reversing your prediabetes—and perhaps even produce a remission if you already have type 2 diabetes—by following the strategies in this book. If you're taking diabetes medications or daily insulin injections, you can reduce your required dosage by using these strategies to improve your glucose control and enhance your body's insulin sensitivity. In either case, you'll be reversing your direction on the diabetes pathway.

The Three Stages of the Diabetes Pathway

STAGE 1: EARLY INSULIN RESISTANCE

In this stage, the body's insulin-dependent tissues—particularly the skeletal muscles, which are where most of your blood glucose is metabolized—have lost some of their ability to respond to insulin. The fat tissues, which also need insulin in order to metabolize glucose, and the liver, which shuts down glucose production when stimulated by insulin, are both affected during early insulin resistance as well. Glucose levels may be normal at this stage, but the pancreas has begun producing insulin in greater amounts to overcome the difficulties of processing glucose on the cellular level. Because fasting blood glucose tests and even oral glucose tolerance tests can produce normal results in this stage, the best way to determine whether your insulin sensitivity is impaired is to check for elevated insulin levels.

The Diabetes Reset **promise:** Insulin sensitivity can typically be restored to normal by employing the Diabetes Reset strategies at this stage.

STAGE 2A: PREDIABETES/IMPAIRED GLUCOSE TOLERANCE

Defined as having a glucose level of 140 mg/dL to 190 mg/dL two hours after taking a 75-gram oral glucose tolerance test, this prediabetic state is a more advanced state of insulin resistance. Not only are insulin levels elevated, but insulin production is beginning to fall short of what's needed to metabolize a large load of blood glucose—a sign that the beta cells of the pancreas are starting to fail. Interventions in the form of healthier nutrition, exercise, and weight loss are critical at this point to avoid the development of diabetes and the need for medications.

The Diabetes Reset **promise:** By following the Diabetes Reset strategies at this stage, you not only can avoid the need for medication for prediabetes (which of course comes with side effects) but you can also prevent the development of type 2 diabetes.

STAGE 2B: PREDIABETES/IMPAIRED FASTING GLUCOSE

Defined as a glucose level of 100 mg/dL to 125 mg/dL on a fasting glucose test, at this stage insulin resistance and pancreas failure have progressed to the point where insulin production can't keep up with the pressure to metabolize glucose even when the blood glucose level is low. Diabetes medication is frequently prescribed at this stage.

The Diabetes Reset **promise:** As with impaired glucose tolerance, if you aggressively employ the strategies outlined in this book at this stage, you can still avoid the need for medication and prevent the development of type 2 diabetes.

STAGE 3: TYPE 2 DIABETES

Type 2 diabetes is considered to have set in when fasting blood glucose levels are consistently 126 mg/dL or higher and oral glucose tolerance test results are consistently above 200 mg/dL. At this stage, blood glucose levels are dangerously high and will begin causing serious damage to health if steps aren't taken to control them with medication and other approaches.

The Diabetes Reset **promise:** If you have been diagnosed with type 2 diabetes, the Diabetes Reset strategies will enable you to control your diabetes more easily and effectively, and may also allow you to "reset" your need for medications since in many cases type 2 diabetes can be successfully controlled by a combination of healthy nutrition, exercise, and maintenance of a normal weight as measured by body mass index (BMI). Of course, you must discuss your plan with your doctor, and you should never stop taking medication without consulting with your doctor.

The Diabetes Reset Message: Hope, Optimism, and Opportunity

No one *wants* to hear the news that their blood glucose isn't what it should be. If, however, you are among the hundreds of millions of people around the globe with either prediabetes or type 2 diabetes, I encourage you to look at this moment as an opportunity to begin taking strides toward better health and a vastly improved glucose metabolism and fat metabolism. We know that most of the underlying causes of prediabetes and type 2 diabetes can be improved, and your body's glucose metabolism reset to a more normal level, by following the evidence-based strategies in *The Diabetes Reset*. The message this book brings is one of hope—based on the knowledge that the ability to improve your health and well-being is now in your hands—and of optimism, because you have already taken the first step toward "resetting" your glucose metabolism and laying the foundation for an active and healthy life.

Five Important Blood Tests You Should Know About

The following five blood tests can all play a part in detecting whether your body is having problems metabolizing blood glucose and regulating fat levels—and, just as important, monitoring the progress of your antidiabetes program.

1. FASTING BLOOD GLUCOSE TEST

This blood test will typically be administered by your primary care physician as part of your annual physical examination. It involves sending a blood sample to a laboratory to measure your blood glucose levels when there is no food in your digestive system. (Typically, people are advised to eat nothing from midnight onward prior to having their blood drawn.) An abnormally high result on this test is often the first sign that someone is having difficulty metabolizing blood glucose or that they already have diabetes.

What the results mean:

- A level under 100 mg/dL is considered normal.

- A level of 100 to 125 mg/dL is an indication of impaired fasting glucose, a sign of prediabetes (and usually insulin resistance as well) that tends to appear sometime after impaired glucose tolerance has set in. A reading in this range indicates that you need to focus intensively on the Diabetes Reset strategies. You might also follow up with an oral glucose tolerance test to confirm the results.

- A level of 126 mg/dL or above indicates that you may have type 2 diabetes. If you have a reading in this range, your doctor may follow up with a second fasting test (two high readings are required for a definitive diagnosis of type 2 diabetes) or an oral glucose tolerance test.

- At times, a nonfasting (or random) glucose test will be given to spot-check blood glucose levels. In this case, any reading above 200 mg/dL is considered a sign of possible diabetes.

2. HEMOGLOBIN A1C TEST

This is another laboratory blood test that is commonly administered as part of your annual physical. It determines average blood glucose levels over the past two to three months by measuring blood levels of hemoglobin A1C—a protein that forms over time from the interaction between hemoglobin and blood glucose. Because this is an ongoing, predictable chemical process, the fraction of A1C in your blood reflects exactly how much glucose your hemoglobin has been exposed to over an extended period, that is, the preceding ninety days. If your blood glucose was normal over this entire period, this fraction will be normal. If your glucose has been elevated for some or all of this extended period, the fraction will be elevated in exact proportion to how much excess blood glucose your hemoglobin was exposed to over this time. So a single blood draw to test for A1C will tell you what your average blood glucose levels were over the past ninety days.

What the results mean:

- A level between 4% and 5.6% is considered normal.

- A level of 5.7% to 6.4% is considered a sign of prediabetes.

- A level of 6.5% or above indicates that you may have type 1 or type 2 diabetes. For people who have been diagnosed with type 1 or 2 diabetes and are being treated for it, the recommended goal is typically to maintain an HA1C reading of 7% or below.

3. ORAL GLUCOSE TOLERANCE TEST

This test measures your body's ability to metabolize glucose. Although typically done to confirm a diagnosis of prediabetes or type 2 diabetes, it can actually detect problems with glucose control earlier than a fasting blood glucose test. One version of this test involves two blood draws (*oral* simply refers to the glucose solution you drink prior to the second blood draw). The first sample is taken after fasting for at least eight hours, after which you will be given a solution to drink containing 75 grams of glucose. Two hours after you drink the solution, another blood sample is taken and analyzed for glucose levels. There is also a three-hour version of this test involving a 100-gram glucose dose and four measurements—fasting, then at one, two, and three hours after drinking the glucose.

What the results of the two-hour test mean:

- A post-ingestion level under 140 mg/dL is considered normal.

- A level from 140 mg/dL to 199 mg/dL is an indication of impaired glucose tolerance, a form of prediabetes that typically means insulin resistance has set in.

- A level of 200 mg/dL or higher indicates that you may have type 2 diabetes. If the test is repeated a second time with the same result, this is considered a definitive diagnosis of type 2 diabetes.

- On the modified screening test for gestational diabetes, a reading above 130 mg/dL is considered elevated. In this case, a three-hour oral glucose tolerance test is administered as a follow-up.

4. INSULIN TEST

This blood test measures the amount of insulin in your blood. Although it is used most often to test for low blood sugar (hypoglycemia), it can also be used to detect early insulin resistance that has not yet progressed to prediabetes. Although blood glucose tests will still yield normal results at this stage of insulin resistance, elevated insulin levels are an indication that your body has to produce more insulin to keep your blood glucose in a normal range. Your insulin test results can be evaluated on their own or combined mathematically with your glucose test results using an approach called a homeostatic model assessment (HOMA) to assess whether you have insulin resistance.

What the results mean:

- A level from 5 µU/mL to 20 µU/mL (microunits per milliliter) is considered normal at fasting.

- A level above 20 µU/mL at fasting is an indication that you may have hyperinsulinemia—a sign that your pancreas is producing more insulin than normal to compensate for insulin resistance.

5. BLOOD GLUCOSE MONITORING

Regular glucose monitoring is routinely recommended for people with type 1 and type 2 diabetes in order to keep track of their blood glucose levels. Those with mild type 2 diabetes may check their glucose once a day, whereas those with type 1 and advanced type 2 diabetes may check it several times or more daily, including an hour after meals, to check on how well their insulin medications are working. I recommend that people with prediabetes or mild type 2 diabetes also monitor their blood glucose several times a day for a period of time while implementing the strategies in *The Diabetes Reset*. That way you can begin to get an idea of how your body is responding to the different approaches outlined in this book. A number of good, inexpensive home glucose monitoring kits are available. To test your blood glucose, you simply insert a disposable test strip into the accompanying meter, then prick your finger and dab a drop of blood onto the strip. Your blood glucose level will appear on the meter's display within seconds.

What the results mean:
Because blood glucose levels measured this way will vary from person to person, what is most important is how your blood glucose levels change from one reading to the next. If a reading is higher than usual at a particular time of day, this indicates problems with glucose control. If your readings drop consistently over time, it's a sign that your Diabetes Reset strategies are working.

Monitoring Your Health as You Go

As you implement the Diabetes Reset strategies, it is also essential that you continue to monitor your overall health, including your blood glucose status, and keep a careful watch for potential complications related to elevated blood glucose levels. The following chart is a one-year medical checklist, outlining all the key diabetes-related tests and examinations you should undergo during any given year. I recommend downloading and printing this chart (you can find it at: workman .com/thediabetesreset) and keeping it where you can reference it easily. I also recommend sharing this checklist with your doctor to make sure you're both on the same page regarding your medical care.

CHECKLIST FOR YOUR DIABETES CARE

TESTS/EXAMS	USUAL GOAL	HOW OFTEN	MY RESULT	DATE
A1C test	<7%	Every 3–6 months		
Total cholesterol	<200 mg/dL (5.2 mmol/L)	Once a year		
LDL cholesterol	<100 mg/dL (2.6 mmol/L)	Once a year		
HDL cholesterol	Male: >40 mg/dL (1.0 mmol/L) Female: >50 mg/dL (1.3 mmol/L)	Once a year		
Triglycerides (TG)	<150 mg/dL (1.7 mmol/L)	Once a year		
Urine microalbumin	<30 mcg/mg (mcg/mg creatinine)	Once a year		
Dilated eye exam	Early detection	Once a year		
Foot exam	Early detection	Every 3–6 months		
Foot exam—self-check	Early detection	Every day		
Blood pressure	<130/80	Every 3–6 months		
Waist circumference	Male: <102 cm (40 inches)* Female: <88 cm (35 inches)*	Every medical visit		
BMI	<25**	Every medical visit		
Stress test	Early detection	Discuss with your health-care provider***		
Flu shots	Early prevention	Once a year		

* Asian American and Asian males should aim for <90 cm (35.5 inches). Asian American and Asian females should aim for <80 cm (31.5 inches).

** Asian Americans and Asians should aim for <24.

*** If you: complain of typical or atypical chest pain
   have an abnormal electrocardiography (ECG)
   have a diagnosis of peripheral artery disease or carotid disease
   are >35 years of age with a sedentary lifestyle and are about to start a rigorous exercise program

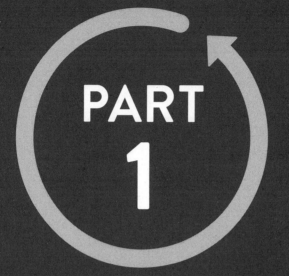

PART 1

THE DIABETES RESET TOOLBOX:

Eight Essential Strategies
for Preventing and Controlling
Type 2 Diabetes

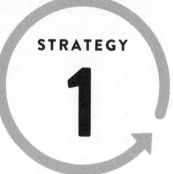

STRATEGY

1

THE RURAL ASIAN DIET (RAD) EATING PLAN: CUT YOUR FAT INTAKE IN HALF AND DOUBLE YOUR FIBER

Large-scale population studies and a groundbreaking clinical trial at the Joslin Diabetes Center have shown that insulin sensitivity, glucose metabolism, and type 2 diabetes risk can all be significantly improved by switching to a low-fat, high-fiber diet consisting of 70% carbohydrates, 15% fat, and 15% protein, including 15 grams of dietary fiber for every 1,000 calories consumed. This chapter provides detailed information on how to implement this dietary approach, known as the Rural Asian Diet (RAD) eating plan.

Key findings:

- The amount of fat you eat and your total calorie consumption— rather than carbohydrate consumption—are what drive the development of obesity, insulin resistance, and type 2 diabetes.

- A diet consisting mainly of high-fiber carbohydrates is associated with weight loss, improved insulin action, enhanced glucose control, and reduced risk of type 2 diabetes.

everal years ago, fifty households across the Boston metropolitan area began getting some very special deliveries, courtesy of the Joslin Diabetes Center. The recipients, all of whom were at high risk for developing type 2 diabetes due to their family history or a diagnosis of prediabetes or glucose intolerance, had been selected to participate in Joslin's Asian Diet Study, a clinical research project testing a new antidiabetes diet based on traditional Asian eating patterns. For eight weeks, we sent each of them a series of prepared breakfasts, lunches, dinners, and snacks on a near-daily basis. The meals all had one thing in common: They were very low in fat, and rich in high-fiber grains, vegetables, and fruits.

The study participants enjoyed the food and had no problem sticking to the diet. More important, at the end of the eight weeks, every one of them showed significant improvement in their insulin sensitivity. Many of them showed improvements in their glucose tolerance as well. The subjects also all improved their cholesterol profiles, and almost all lost weight, even though we adjusted the calories in an attempt to prevent them from losing weight.

The meals we were feeding these Boston residents were based on an eating plan known as the Rural Asian Diet, or RAD for short. It is the diet that people across Asia—and around the world, for that matter—have thrived on for many centuries. It is also a diet that is rapidly vanishing from the planet as more and more people shift to the eating pattern that many people in the Western hemisphere (and a growing number in the Eastern hemisphere) now follow: getting more than one third of their calories from fat and supplementing that with mostly refined carbohydrates that contain just a fraction of the fiber in the Rural Asian Diet.

This high-fat, low-fiber Western diet has the reverse effect of the Rural Asian Diet: When people eat it, they gain weight and their risk of diabetes goes up. You can see the effects all around you: Two thirds of adult Americans are now overweight or obese, at least 26 million Americans have type 2 diabetes, and another 86 million have prediabetes, meaning they're on the way to developing diabetes unless they change course and start eating differently.

Introducing the Rural Asian Diet

One of the first questions asked by people who have just been diagnosed with prediabetes or type 2 diabetes is, what should I be eating? In this chapter, I will outline a high-fiber, low-fat diet that you can follow with full confidence. It will increase your insulin sensitivity and glucose control, improve your underlying risk factors for diabetes, and help you maintain a healthy weight—all without any specific limits on the amount of calories you consume. If you adopt the healthy eating pattern described in this chapter, you will also be lowering your risk of cardiovascular disease and certain cancers, and you may possibly lose weight. Plus, you'll feel terrific too!

At the Joslin Asian Clinic, we call this dietary approach the Rural Asian Diet (RAD) eating plan because it mirrors the nutritional mix that East Asian populations have lived and thrived on for centuries. The term *rural* is used to distinguish it from a more recent dietary trend that has taken root in the urban centers of China, India, Thailand, Korea, and other Asian nations. Whereas the Rural Asian Diet is low in fat and high in dietary fiber and complex, unrefined carbohydrates, the modern urban Asian diet is very similar to the diet most Americans consume—high in fat and low in fiber, with a large percentage of carbohydrates coming from processed foods such as white flour, white rice, and sugar.

Why the Rural Asian Diet Is Right for You

In addition to its benefits in terms of improving insulin sensitivity and other diabetes risk factors, our research shows that the RAD eating plan is a diet that people are able to stick to. For one thing, the Rural Asian Diet doesn't call for restricting the amount of calories you consume, unless you decide to embark on the type of time-limited weight-loss program outlined in the next chapter. And although we advise minimizing fat and animal protein intake and using low-fat or unsaturated fat alternatives whenever possible, the Rural Asian Diet does not require that you become a vegetarian or totally avoid red meat or dairy products. The Rural Asian Diet *does* encourage you to eat as many healthy, high-fiber, complex carbohydrate foods as you can and to choose low-fat alternatives whenever possible. When you do this, you will find that you naturally begin to cut back on high-fat and low-fiber foods.

The Rural Asian Diet is also not an "all or nothing" proposition. We believe—and evidence suggests—that the diet's mix of 70% carbs, 15% protein, and 15% fat, with at least 15 grams of dietary fiber per 1,000 calories, is the best ratio for your health and glucose profile. But even if you use the guidelines in this chapter to make only modest changes in terms of cutting fat intake and boosting daily intake of dietary fiber, you will be taking an important step toward improving your glucose control and rolling back your prediabetes or diabetes.

Finally, the RAD eating plan is fun to eat. In our posttrial surveys, all of the subjects in our study indicated that they found the diet satisfying and enjoyable.

Debunking the Media: Why Dietary Fat Is Not the Key to Good Health, Carbs Are Not All Bad, and Sugar Is Not the Root of All Evil

One of the big challenges today in trying to promote an evidence-based approach to preventing and controlling diabetes is that so many health "experts" are misrepresenting scientific knowledge to push ideas that make for great sound bites but that actually do more harm than good to people's health. In this chapter and the two that follow, I'll do my best to debunk some of these ideas that have gained the most popular attention.

MEDIA MYTH: EATING TOO MANY CARBS IS THE REASON AMERICANS ARE OVERWEIGHT.

The problem with this concept is that it throws out the baby with the bath water. It's true that Americans are eating too many refined carbohydrates, including white flour and sugar, that contain empty calories—which is to say, they provide energy but little else in the form of nutrients. But as I'll discuss in this chapter, there are plenty of other carbohydrate-rich foods—whole grains, legumes, vegetables, and fruits—that not only contain a huge variety of health-promoting phytonutrients (nutrients derived from plants) but are also high in dietary fiber, which has been strongly linked to improved glucose metabolism and decreased diabetes risk. In fact, studies suggest that a diet high in fiber and complex (nonrefined) carbohydrates is the healthiest diet you could possibly eat.

This is not to say that a low-carb diet won't help you lose weight. Many people have lost weight in the short term through this approach, which involves combining total caloric restriction with a particular restriction on carbohydrate intake for several months in order to force the body to start burning its fat stores as fuel instead of glucose (which is derived from carbs). A low-carb diet is not a healthy, sustainable diet over the long term, however, for reasons I'll discuss at length in this chapter.

MEDIA MYTH: AMERICA'S OBESITY AND DIABETES EPIDEMICS ARE COMPLETELY DUE TO OVERCONSUMPTION OF SUGAR AND FRUCTOSE.

This view, which has been promoted heavily by quite a few health experts, has an element of truth to it. There is no question that Americans eat too much of these sweeteners, and there is also no question that fructose—which makes up half of sucrose (table sugar) and about 55% of high-fructose corn syrup, widely used to sweeten soft drinks and other food products—is singularly bad for your health. In fact, fructose is actually a fat masquerading as a carbohydrate because it is digested differently than other carbohydrates, being converted into fatty acids by the liver instead of being broken down into glucose. It's also fairly clear that consuming too much sugar and fructose, especially in the form of soda, is a significant part of why Americans are overweight. But a significant percentage of people can—and do—become overweight and develop type 2 diabetes even though they *aren't* consuming large amounts of sugar and fructose. The real villain here is an old and decidedly unsexy one: People are simply eating more calories than they used to. In fact, if you look at USDA data on Americans' food intake from 1970 to 2010, you'll see that while total daily calorie intake for the average American adult went up by 460 calories per day, the amount of daily calories consumed in the form of added sugars stayed largely flat. There's also very little evidence to support another of the claims against fructose, that eating it actually increases (rather than decreases) appetite—in fact, most studies indicate the opposite.

Over this same period of time, survey evidence also indicates that the amount of physical activity Americans get each day actually declined—meaning that these extra 460 daily calories were destined for the body's fat stores. I make these points because, although I certainly encourage everyone to cut back on their intake of these sweeteners, I also don't want you to think that all of your health problems will be solved simply by eliminating them from your diet. In the final analysis, lowering your diabetes risk by losing weight requires cutting back not just on added sugars but on total calories consumed.

MEDIA MYTH: INSULIN PRODUCTION, TRIGGERED BY EATING CARBOHYDRATES, IS WHAT IS CAUSING AMERICANS TO BE OVERWEIGHT.

This myth is related to the "carbs are the enemy" myth. It is based on the fact that one of insulin's actions in the body is to stimulate the body's fat stores to take up fatty acids from the bloodstream and store them, as well as the observation that people who are overweight typically have elevated insulin levels. (The observation that people with diabetes often gain weight when they begin taking insulin medication may have contributed to this concept, although in fact this weight gain is usually due to a combination of rehydrating the body—after it had been dehydrated from elevated glucose levels—and eating too much—after it was nutritionally deprived—also from elevated glucose levels.)

Actual scientific experiments suggest otherwise, however: In a number of studies of mice who were genetically altered so that their insulin levels were several times higher than normal, the altered mice did not gain weight. The fact that obesity causes the fat stores to become insulin resistant—and thus less responsive to insulin's fat-promoting properties—also works against this theory. Scientists have actually found that obesity tends to make the body's fat stores release fatty acids into the bloodstream more readily, which contributes to insulin resistance in the muscles and liver as well. The thinking now is that obesity is the cause of elevated insulin levels rather than the other way around.

MEDIA MYTH: A HIGH-FAT DIET IS THE KEY TO GOOD HEALTH.

This is a particularly frustrating myth to deal with. A number of popular health experts have seized on this idea with almost religious fervor, but the evidence from many large-scale studies clearly links high-fat diets—particularly diets high in saturated fats—with increased risk of weight gain, type 2 diabetes, cardiovascular disease, and certain cancers. One fact that the pro-fat group loves to cite is that the percentage of fat in Americans' diets went down from 1970 to 2000, a period when obesity rates soared and when the antidietary fat message was gaining steam. "America stopped eating fat and got fat," they like to say. But as I'll discuss later in this chapter, national survey data show that the total grams of daily fat consumed by the average American remained virtually unchanged during that time—so any suggestion that Americans somehow cut down on their fat intake over that period is patently false.

Again, it's certainly possible to lose weight in the short term by following a low-carb, high-fat diet so long as total calories are restricted at the same time—but continuing to eat a high-fat diet over a period of years is a recipe for making yourself sick.

The Case for the Rural Asian Diet—How Carbohydrates Got Wrongly Tagged as the Nutritional "Bad Guy"

Let me state right up front that the diet outlined in this chapter will be controversial to some people. That's because the Rural Asian Diet derives the vast majority if its calories—more than two thirds—from carbohydrates. In the world of diabetes medicine, many experts advise people with diabetes or prediabetes to restrict the amount of carbohydrates they eat. The American Diabetes Association (ADA) website, for example, recommends a "moderate carbohydrate" diet in which 45% to 50% of daily calories come from carbohydrates. Some popular diet programs recommend even lower levels of carbohydrates. The developers of the Metabolic Diet, for example, suggest that people with type 2 diabetes try a diet containing just 25% carbohydrates as a starting point, then begin reducing the carb intake from there.

In addition to restricting overall carbohydrate intake, many experts also recommend that people with diabetes or prediabetes limit the amount of carbohydrates they take in at any one time as well—an approach known as carbohydrate counting. The reasoning behind both of these approaches is the same: Carbohydrates are by far the largest dietary source of blood glucose. Because people with prediabetes or diabetes don't metabolize glucose effectively, reducing overall glucose production—including the surge in blood glucose that occurs after eating—means there will be less glucose in your bloodstream to metabolize. This in turn means it should make it easier to keep blood glucose levels under control because you'll require less of your body's own insulin or diabetes medication to keep your blood glucose under control.

This viewpoint, however, is based on a diet high in refined carbohydrates, which has become ubiquitous in modern America. If you consume a majority of complex carbohydrates that are high in fiber, such as whole-grain flour, brown rice, legumes, and vegetables, as outlined in the RAD eating plan, then the carbohydrates you eat will be converted into blood glucose much more slowly, avoiding a blood glucose spike.

Other Faulty Arguments for Restricting Carbs

A number of studies have shown that restricting carbohydrates can also produce rapid weight loss in the short term because the lack of available glucose forces the body to burn its fat stores instead, a process called ketosis. As a result, the "low-carb" approach to eating, as exemplified by the Atkins Diet, has gained a great deal of popularity over the past two decades as a dieting tool.

This trend has been amplified by mounting research on the harmful health effects of simple carbohydrates, including sucrose (table sugar) and high-fructose corn syrup, both widely used as sweeteners in processed foods, and refined flour, another widely used ingredient in commercial food production. Thanks to this combination of factors, carbohydrates have become a dietary villain in many people's eyes.

My own view, however, is that the prevailing advice to restrict overall intake of carbohydrates is misguided and ultimately harmful. It's certainly true that the consumption of processed carbohydrates, especially sugar and fructose (which, by the way, is partly converted into fats by your digestive tract), poses a serious health danger. Most notably, soft drinks containing high-fructose corn syrup appear to be playing a contributory role in America's obesity epidemic. But the scientific evidence simply doesn't support the idea that carbohydrates, as a nutrient category, are the primary cause of our modern diabetes epidemic, particularly when the carbohydrates you consume are mainly complex, nonrefined carbs, high in fiber and rich in phytonutrients—both of which reduce insulin resistance while protecting the health of your pancreas.

The real villain, as I'll discuss in a moment, is dietary fat and its corollary, the excessive amount of total calories that Americans consume on a daily basis. In fact, when our carbohydrate consumption is reduced, fat (which has more than twice as many calories per gram than carbs) is inevitably the nutrient that we start eating more of.

EIGHT REASONS WHY CUTTING BACK ON CARBS IS NOT A GOOD LONG-TERM DIETARY APPROACH

1 Because human beings' protein intake tends to remain remarkably constant (in part because high-protein meals expand more inside the digestive system), cutting back on carbohydrates invariably means eating more fat—which is proven to contribute to insulin resistance, pancreas damage, obesity, systemic inflammation, and cardiovascular disease.

2 Americans' fat intake is already very high. In fact, the so-called antifat era that anticarb advocates keep citing never really happened. Americans consume almost exactly as many grams of fat per day now as they did forty years ago.

3 Eating the right kind of carbs—complex carbohydrates that are high in fiber, including whole grains, vegetables, legumes, and fruit—has

been shown to significantly improve insulin sensitivity, moderate the body's glucose production, leave you more satiated after eating, and reduce the amount of calories your body absorbs from the food you eat.

4 Although a low-carb diet may facilitate weight loss in some individuals by increasing the body's reliance on burning fat stores for energy, health experts agree that this approach should be followed for only a limited time—six to twelve months at most—and that over the long term a low-carb diet poses significant health risks. These include the risks of fat consumption listed previously, as well as the potential for vitamin and mineral deficiencies and possible kidney damage.

5 Experts also agree that the health problems that have been potentially associated with carbohydrate consumption, including obesity, are limited strictly to the consumption of refined carbs—white flour, white rice, sugar, high-fructose corn syrup, and to some extent non-whole-grain pasta and potatoes (which despite being nutritious have a high glycemic index, meaning they create a relatively fast rise in blood glucose after eating them). By minimizing these types of carbs and substituting complex carbohydrates for them, you will eliminate any negative long-term effects of carbs and gain all the benefits of a high-fiber diet listed previously—while also avoiding the negative consequences of a high-fat diet.

6 By eating meals that combine a large percentage of complex carbohydrates, which tend to have a low glycemic index, with a modest amount of protein and fat (primarily nonsaturated fat), and by at the same time avoiding overly large portions, you will experience only a moderate blood glucose rise over a relatively long period of time after eating—thereby preventing the blood glucose "spike" after eating that has traditionally been the reason why people with diabetes have been advised to limit the amount of carbs they eat at any given time.

7 Studies also show that by consistently eating a diet high in complex carbohydrates, you will significantly improve your chances of maintaining a healthy weight over the long term.

8 Finally, a diet high in complex, high-fiber carbohydrates and low in fat has been clearly shown to produce the best results in terms of long-term glycemic control for people with prediabetes or diabetes.

Asia's Story: How a Dietary Shift Led to a Diabetes Epidemic

The key role that consuming more dietary fat—which translates into increased daily caloric intake—plays in the progression of type 2 diabetes becomes evident when you look at the link between diabetes and eating patterns globally. In China, a nation I'm very familiar with and visit often, most of the population has eaten essentially the same diet for centuries. That traditional diet consists of 70% carbohydrates— almost all of it from "complex" carbs such as vegetables, legumes, and whole grains, with very few refined carbohydrates in the form of sugar and white flour. Only 15% of their daily calories comes from fat, with the remaining 15% coming in the form of protein. Among the many millions of people who have followed this diet their entire lives, the incidence of type 2 diabetes is remarkably small: In 1980, when most of China's inhabitants still followed this type diet, the overall diabetes rate for the nation was just 1%.

Since then, a major demographic shift has occurred in China, as millions of people have left their rural, agriculture-based way of life behind and relocated to urban areas. In the process, they've traded their traditional diet for one much closer to what's known as the "typical Western diet." Compared to their rural diet, this Western diet contains an equal percentage of protein (approximately 15% of total calories) but only about 50% of its calories come from carbohydrates—the amount recommended by the ADA, as you'll recall—while 35% of daily calorie intake comes from dietary fat, on average. And because it also contains more simple carbohydrates and fewer complex carbs, the typical Western diet also contains only about one third as much fiber as the traditional rural Asian diet.

During the same time this demographic shift has been occurring, China's diabetes rate has been skyrocketing. According to the most recent data, the percentage of Chinese with diabetes now stands at 11.6%—a more than tenfold increase in just over thirty years! A similarly sharp increase in diabetes has been seen in India, Korea, Indonesia, and Thailand, as well as in second- and third-generation Asian Americans—all of whom have gone through a similar transition from a high-carbohydrate, high-fiber diet to a moderate-carb, low-fiber (and high-fat and high-calorie!) diet. Likewise, a shift from uniform leanness to an increasing incidence of obesity has been observed in recent decades in African cultures that have traditionally consumed a high-carbohydrate diet as high-fat food sources become more available to wealthier individuals.

As an Asian American and a diabetes researcher, I've always taken a strong interest in the treatment and prevention of type 2 diabetes among both Asians and Americans of Asian descent. I'm often asked to speak at gatherings of Asian diabetes experts, and every year I travel to China, Japan, and other Asian countries—where type 2 diabetes has become a pressing topic—to meet with diabetes researchers and clinicians. As I've pointed out repeatedly to these groups, any time a disease increases this rapidly among a specific population, it's clear that environment is playing a major role, because a few decades is not long enough for any significant genetic changes to take place.

One aspect of this epidemic that grabbed my attention is the fact that it has *not* taken hold in rural parts of Asia, where people continue to eat much the same way their ancestors did. In regions where this traditional rural Asian diet is followed, the type 2 diabetes rates are still around 1% to 2%—this, despite their consuming an amount of daily carbohydrates that's well above the amount recommended by the ADA.

As I pondered this fact, I began to speculate that this explosion of type 2 diabetes in Asia (and among Asian Americans) could be related, at least in part, to the fact that Asian populations have increasingly been exchanging traditional rural life for an urban lifestyle—and, in the process, switching from their centuries-old rural Asian diet to a Western-type diet. There is evidence that Asians are more susceptible to type 2 diabetes than other populations and that their risk level for the disease increases substantially with a relatively small weight gain compared to other groups. So perhaps this change in eating patterns was enough to impair the glucose metabolism of a sizeable percentage of this population and cause its recent surge in diabetes rates.

The more I thought about this link, the more plausible it seemed. To test this theory, my Joslin colleagues and I decided to construct a study that would directly measure the impact of these two diets. We wanted to see just how much a high-fat, low-fiber diet might be contributing to the modern epidemic of diabetes and whether this trend could be reversed by a diet that sharply reduces fat intake while significantly boosting people's consumption of dietary fiber.

What About America?

One major piece of evidence cited by the "fat isn't so bad for you" school is that from 1970 to 2006, when the proportion of Americans who are obese grew from about 14% to 32%, Americans also reduced their fat intake slightly when measured as a portion of their total daily calories, from 37% to 34%, and increased their carbohydrate portion from 44% to 49%.

Before jumping to the conclusion that "carbs are making America fat," however, consider this: That percentage decline in calories derived from fat *wasn't* because we were eating less fat. In fact, the total daily amount of fat consumed by the average American went *up* slightly over that period. The percentage went down only because Americans were eating more calories overall.

There's no question that more Americans are eating too many calories, including too many refined, low-fiber carbohydrates: As I note in the next chapter, average portion sizes in America have gotten steadily larger over the past few decades, and many Americans are also now getting far more calories from soft drinks sweetened with high-fructose corn syrup. But I also believe that the foundation for America's obesity and diabetes epidemics already existed, in the form of a diet consisting of one-third fat. As Americans became less physically active and began adding several hundred extra calories per day, mostly in the form of refined carbohydrates, that was enough to tip millions of people's metabolisms further toward obesity, insulin resistance, and, for a vulnerable subgroup, type 2 diabetes.

Heroes and Villains: How Dietary Fat Helps Cause Type 2 Diabetes and How Dietary Fiber Helps Prevent It

Joslin's Asian Diet Study was one of the first prospective studies to look at the benefits of a high-fiber, very low-fat diet for people at risk for type 2 diabetes. There is, however, already a large body of research supporting the idea that a consistently high-fat diet *contributes significantly* to the development of insulin resistance, prediabetes, and type 2 diabetes in a variety of ways. In fact, when scientists want to induce insulin resistance in a laboratory animal, the standard approach is to feed it a high-fat diet!

At the same time, there is clear evidence that a high-fiber diet can dramatically improve insulin sensitivity in a relatively short time and that in the long run it *lowers* type 2 diabetes risk significantly. Here is a summary of what this research is showing:

HOW DIETARY FAT INCREASES INSULIN RESISTANCE AND TYPE 2 DIABETES RISK

A high-fat diet makes it easier to gain weight and keep it on. Both human population studies and animal studies consistently show that a high-fat diet is more likely to promote obesity, which is a primary risk factor for prediabetes and type 2 diabetes. One key reason for this is fat's high energy density: 1 gram of fat contains 9 calories, whereas 1 gram of carbohydrate or protein contains just 4 calories. There is evidence suggesting that this, combined with the palatability of fat, makes it easier to consume more calories than you actually need when eating a high-fat meal. There is also evidence that once someone becomes obese, his or her body tends to store dietary fat as fat tissue more readily rather than use it for fuel—making it harder to lose excess body fat through energy expenditure.

High dietary fat intake directly reduces insulin sensitivity in the muscles and liver.
A high-fat diet is associated with increased levels of free fatty acids (FFAs) in the bloodstream, which in turn appear to induce insulin resistance in the muscles—preventing them from metabolizing glucose effectively—and in the liver, where it causes increased glucose production. These insulin-blunting effects appear to be due to both disruption of insulin signaling activity by certain fatty acid components and to inflammatory activity triggered by these fatty acids. (See box on page 39: How a Single High-Fat Meal Can Impair Your Insulin Sensitivity.)

A high-fat diet damages the pancreas.
Recent animal studies have found that when mice were fed a high-fat diet for a number of months in what would be their "middle-aged" years, they developed inflammation in a part of the pancreas called the islets of Langerhans—a condition that is a known risk factor for type 2 diabetes. The mice also had reduced insulin production and elevated blood glucose levels. Earlier animal studies found that a high-fat diet also inhibits expression of a key gene in the pancreas that is involved in insulin production.

A high-fat diet during pregnancy may increase diabetes risk for offspring.
When obesity-resistant rats were fed a high-fat diet during pregnancy, it affected gene expression in the livers of their unborn offspring, causing their livers to overproduce glucose after birth.

Diets high in fat can cause the bacterial flora in the intestinal tracts to change in a way that increases inflammation in the body, contributing to insulin resistance and diabetes.
A recent report showed that changing from a vegetarian diet to one high in meat and fat will increase the amount of gut flora that are bile toler-ant. These bile-tolerant bacteria have been linked to the development of inflammatory bowel disease (an inflammation of the intestines), which can cause systemwide insulin resistance, much as obesity can. These changes induced by substantially increasing fat intake help explain how a Western diet can promote type 2 diabetes.

HOW FIBER IMPROVES YOUR GLUCOSE METABOLISM
Dietary fiber enhances your ability to metabolize blood glucose in a number of different ways—some of which have been known for many years and others that were discovered only recently. Here are some of the key antidiabetes benefits of a high-fiber diet:

Dietary fiber directly improves insulin sensitivity.
A number of studies, including our own, have found that eating more dietary fiber for a period of weeks or months is linked to a reduction in biomarkers for insulin resistance. This may be due in part to dietary fiber's anti-inflammatory effects—high-fiber diets have been associated with reduced blood levels of C-reactive protein, a marker for systemic inflammation—and also to the fact that the short-chain fatty acids that fiber produces when it ferments in the intestinal tract tend to inhibit the breakdown of the body's fat stores into free fatty acids. As we'll see in the next chapter, this breakdown of fat stores appears to play a major role in creating insulin resistance in the skeletal muscles. In addition, the intestinal fermentation of fiber—particularly insoluble fiber—has been shown to stimulate production of glucose in the intes-tines themselves, which triggers a reaction in the body that makes it more responsive to insulin.

How a Single High-Fat Meal
Can Impair Your Insulin Sensitivity

It is well known that eating carbohydrates causes a rise in glucose levels afterward. But what many people don't realize is that a high-fat meal can increase glucose levels as well, by increasing the level of FFAs in the bloodstream. *FFA* stands for "free fatty acid." Free fatty acids circulate through the bloodstream when fat stores are broken down to provide energy—which typically happens overnight, when blood glucose levels are low and an additional energy supply is needed. Normally, FFA levels then drop quite low during the day, as you resume eating and your body starts burning more glucose again.

The problem occurs when blood levels of FFAs become abnormally elevated—a situation shown to play a direct role in causing insulin resistance both in the skeletal muscles (where they impair the ability of the muscles to take up and utilize blood glucose) and in the liver (where they cause the liver to produce more glucose than normal). People who are overweight or obese appear to have chronically higher FFA levels than people who are lean, particularly if they have a large amount of abdominal fat. But FFA levels in the blood will also rise after a high-fat meal, if the amount of the dietary fat you eat exceeds your body's ability to convert that fat into stored fat tissue.

Studies have shown that elevated FFA levels in the blood can cause signs of insulin resistance within two to four hours. Because postmealtime is when glucose levels are already elevated, the result is an extra fat-induced rise in blood glucose. If you are routinely eating high-fat meals, of course, this increase in insulin resistance and resulting rise in blood glucose becomes an ongoing affair.

Elevated FFA levels, similar to elevated glucose levels, can also cause damage to the blood vessels, especially the endothelial cells (the cells lining your blood vessels). The reason: Elevated FFAs can cause the endothelial cells to become sticky. Circulating white blood cells then adhere to them and become activated, causing inflammation of the blood vessels. This inflammation in turn accelerates the process of atherosclerosis (hardening of the arteries), which is the leading cause of heart disease in diabetic patients.

Interestingly, studies have also found that suppressing FFA levels for just twelve hours is enough to significantly improve insulin sensitivity in both people with type 2 diabetes and nondiabetic people—suggesting that if you switch to a low-fat diet, you will see immediate improvements in your own ability to metabolize blood glucose.

Because dietary fiber is digested more slowly, glucose is released more slowly into the bloodstream after eating a high-fiber meal.

Soluble fiber's general effect of slowing down the digestive process means that the carbohydrates we eat take longer to be broken down into glucose. As a result, the release of glucose into the blood after eating tends to occur more slowly over a longer period of time following a high-fiber meal. This means that glucose doesn't rise to as high a peak after eating, putting less stress on the glucose metabolism process.

Fiber signals the liver to manufacture less glucose.

Finally, the same fermentation process that signals the body to become more responsive to insulin also suppresses glucose production in the liver—countering the liver's glucose overproduction that occurs as the result of insulin resistance.

A diet high in fiber makes you feel more satisfied compared to eating the same amount of calories in low-fiber foods, making it easier to eat less.

A number of studies have found that people who eat diets high in fiber feel more "full" after eating and also feel less hungry between meals. This has been demonstrated both in subjects on calorie-restricted diets and in people who were able to eat as much food as they wanted.

Fiber increases satiety (the feeling that you've had enough to eat) in several ways: For starters, dietary fiber is simply bulkier than other nutrients. This causes the stomach to become more distended when you eat fiber, which sends appetite-suppressing signals to the brain. Soluble fiber also slows down the passage of food through the digestive tract, causing nutrients to be absorbed more slowly, which has been linked to an increase in digestion-related sensations of satiety. There is also evidence that the need to chew high-fiber foods more thoroughly than other food types contributes to a feeling of being full. Finally, fiber also appears to act directly on cells in the intestinal wall to trigger a hormonal response that may contribute to feelings of satiety.

In addition, foods high in fiber are generally lower in calories, period. Because research shows that we judge how much to eat based on the actual volume of food we consume, this effect should also tend to reduce the amount of calories you take in.

Dietary fiber reduces fat intake and also alters your intestinal microbiome so that it consumes more calories.
It is also thought that a high-fiber diet may contribute to lower body weight by slowing the digestion and absorption of dietary fat, so that fewer fat calories are consumed by the body. There is also evidence that a high-fiber diet alters the makeup of the gut microbiome (the many billions of bacteria and other microbes that populate the intestinal tract) in a way that causes these microbes to consume more calories from the food that you eat, again allowing fewer calories to pass into the body.

A high-fiber diet makes it easier to maintain a healthy weight.
The points that a diet high in fiber results in increased satiety and an altered intestinal microbiome both suggest that a high-fiber diet can help prevent excess body fat. And in fact, a number of studies have confirmed that the more fiber people eat, the lower their body weight and body fat tends to be. In addition, several short-term studies of overweight people on high-fiber diets have found that these diets tend to result in moderate weight loss. As we'll see in the next chapter, losing even a relatively small amount of weight will improve insulin sensitivity and reduce type 2 diabetes risk.

Still, the antidiabetes effects of a high-fiber diet, as found in our Rural Asian Diet Study and similar clinical trials, appear to be greater than can be explained through the amount of weight lost by the study subjects. This suggests that fiber helps prevent diabetes through other mechanisms as well.

Putting the Rural Asian Diet to the Test

At Joslin, our interest in the Rural Asian Diet goes back almost two decades. It is linked closely to our interest in finding ways to combat the growing diabetes epidemic among Asian Americans, who are

There Are No Specific Calorie Restrictions on the Rural Asian Diet

As I mentioned earlier, one of the attractive aspects of the Rural Asian Diet eating plan is that *unless you're on a targeted weight-loss program*, you can eat as many calories as you want—provided you stay within the diet's nutritional guidelines—with a good chance that you won't gain any weight. In fact, you may even lose some excess pounds.

In our Rural Asian Diet Study, we strongly encouraged our subjects to eat more than they were, because they were actively losing weight over their eight weeks on the diet. That was exactly what we *didn't* want to happen because our aim was to measure effects on insulin sensitivity and glucose control independent of weight loss. Yet they consistently told us they couldn't eat any more than they were because the high-fiber foods in their diet were making them feel full.

Their weight loss wasn't entirely due to feeling satiated from the fiber, however. That was proven when our subjects shifted to a high-fat Western diet in the middle of our study: Eating exactly the same amount of calories as they were before, they switched direction and started *gaining* weight rather than losing.

almost twice as likely as the general U.S. population to develop type 2 diabetes. This is partly due to a genetic vulnerability—but when you look at the traditionally low rates in Asian Americans' countries of origin, it's clear that environment, and diet in particular, is playing an important part as well.

In order to focus more closely on this problem, Joslin established the Asian American Diabetes Initiative (AADI) in 2000. The AADI runs a clinic where Asian American patients with type 2 diabetes can make appointments with physicians and dietitians and diabetes educators who are culturally sensitive to this population's needs; the clinic also sponsors outreach events designed to help educate Asian Americans about diabetes risk and encourages adoption of a more active lifestyle and healthier eating patterns. I'm happy to report that this approach has dramatically improved the outcomes of patients in the Joslin Asian Clinic. Their glucose, blood pressure, and cholesterol control are all much better than the national average.

In 2006, the Joslin AADI decided to test our hypothesis that the high diabetes rate among Asian Americans is being caused in large part by a mass switch from a rural Asian diet to a typical Western diet, by carrying out a clinical trial that would assess the impact of this dietary shift.

Ultimately, it took us four years at a cost of several million dollars to design and execute a study that would accurately measure the effects of these two dietary approaches. We asked some of Boston's top chefs

The Asian Paradox:
Not Overweight but Still Prone to Diabetes

We embarked on our study of the Rural Asian Diet as an outgrowth of Joslin's Asian American Diabetes Initiative, which was established to help address the high rates of type 2 diabetes among Asian Americans—and now, increasingly, among residents of Asian nations as well. One puzzling aspect of the rising rates of diabetes in people of Asian origin is that they tend to develop impaired glucose tolerance at a relatively lower body weight than other ethnic groups. Although most people in other populations typically start showing signs of insulin resistance when their BMI (a figure obtained by dividing your weight by the square of your height) hits 27, Asians may begin showing indications of insulin resistance with a BMI as low as 23 to 25—a level considered a healthy and normal weight in other ethnic populations.

As of yet, we have no definitive explanation for this difference. Possible reasons include genetic differences in body frame, which result in a larger percentage body fat for a given weight among Asian populations. Asians may also have a greater tendency to develop abdominal fat, which has been shown to have an especially strong association with insulin resistance. It has also been suggested that Asians may have fewer beta cells in their pancreas or are more likely to have beta cell impairment, which would hasten the time when their insulin output can no longer keep up with the increased demand brought on by insulin resistance.

As these factors continue to be investigated, our own Asian Diet Study clearly shows that people of Asian descent are being affected negatively by the typical high-fat, low-fiber Western diet. Our research also demonstrates that Asian individuals who are at high risk for type 2 diabetes can benefit substantially from switching to the Rural Asian Diet—even though the exact cause of the high rate of diabetes among Asian American and Asian populations remains unknown.

to develop ways of preparing high-carb, high-fiber foods in a way that Americans would enjoy eating. After we were satisfied with the culinary quality of meals we were offering, we began recruiting people in the greater Boston area who were at increased risk for type 2 diabetes due to a family history of the disease, a medical history of gestational diabetes, impaired glucose tolerance, or impaired fasting glucose.

We eventually enlisted twenty-eight East Asian Americans as well as twenty-two Caucasian Americans with a similar risk profile. Our theory was that Caucasians would show less impact from a change in diet, being more genetically adapted to the Western mix of nutrients. Once the subjects were recruited, we gave them a comprehensive exam, including analysis of their blood lipids and insulin sensitivity.

Finally, we were ready to begin testing the traditional Asian diet. Forty-one of the subjects from both ethnic populations were placed in our intervention group, who would make the switch from a traditional Asian diet to a typical Western diet midway through the study, while nine subjects were randomly assigned to a control group that would stay on the traditional Asian diet for the duration of the trial.

A registered dietitian helped our chefs create the recipes and menus that we used in the study. The caloric content of each meal was calculated based on the participant's age, weight, height, medical condition, and physical activity. The nutritional content of our traditional Asian diet meals were calibrated so that 70% of their calories came from carbohydrates, 15% from protein, and 15% from fat, with 15 grams of fiber per every 1,000 calories and only a small portion of daily protein intake—just 20%—coming from animal sources. In the typical Western diet that half of the subjects switched to in mid-trial, 50% of the calories came from carbohydrate, 16% of the energy from protein, and 34% of the energy from fat, with 6 grams of fiber per 1,000 calories, and 60% to 80% of protein coming from animal sources.

For sixteen weeks, we shipped three daily meals plus a snack to study subjects across the greater Boston area. Various chefs in the Boston area cooked the meals, and they were delivered to each subject every two to three days to maintain freshness. Participants were instructed to

consume only foods we provided
to them over the course of the
study and were asked to limit their
alcohol consumption. Because we
didn't want them to gain or lose
weight during the study, they were
weighed every two weeks and the
calorie content of their meals was
adjusted accordingly.

We also took additional measurements of our subjects' insulin
sensitivity, blood lipids, and other
key parameters at the beginning
and end of the first eight-week
period, when all of our subjects
were on the RAD eating plan. At
the end of the first eight weeks, our
intervention group was switched
to a typical Western diet for an additional eight weeks, while the control
group continued on the Asian diet. When the second eight-week period
was concluded, the entire cohort underwent lab testing again.

> ## The RAD Eating Plan Versus the Typical Western Diet
>
> ---
>
> **The Rural Asian Diet contains . . .**
> 15% fat
> 70% carbohydrates
> 15% protein (mostly from plant sources)
> 15 grams of fiber per 1,000 calories
>
> **The typical Western diet contains . . .**
> 34% fat
> 50% carbohydrates
> 16% protein (mostly from animal sources)
> 6 grams of fiber per 1,000 calories

All told, forty of our fifty original subjects—seven in the control
group and thirty-three in the intervention group—completed the full
sixteen weeks of the study. We were pleased that everyone who stayed
on in the control and intervention groups stuck faithfully to the Asian
diet during the study period, but we weren't all that surprised: In addition to being carefully taste-tested, the makeup of the traditional Asian
diet, with its 70% carbohydrate content, is one that people find naturally
appealing because our bodies are born to burn carbohydrates.

We also weren't surprised to find that our Asian American subjects
who switched from the Asian diet to the typical Western diet midway
through the study showed a significant decrease in insulin sensitivity after
making the switch. This finding confirmed our theory that the Western
diet was having a negative impact on the Asian populations both in the

United States and in Asia itself. The insulin sensitivity of our Caucasian Americans didn't appear to be affected by the switch back to the Western diet they were accustomed to, although they did show increases in total and LDL cholesterol as well as inflammatory markers.

What we *were* surprised by, though, was the degree to which *both* study populations—Asian Americans and Caucasian Americans—improved their diabetes risk factors after consuming the traditional Asian diet for just eight weeks. Both groups showed significant improvements in insulin sensitivity on the RAD eating plan and also had significant reductions in their total and LDL cholesterol levels. Also surprising was the fact that our study participants lost an average of 3% in body weight on the traditional Asian diet—this, despite our best efforts to *prevent* any weight loss!

The analysis of our data has been completed, and the study has been published. Meanwhile, the implications of our research are clear: The

The RAD Target: 33 Grams of Fat and 30 Grams of Fiber per Day

The Rural Asian Diet is based on keeping fat intake low—around 15% of total daily calories—and fiber intake high, in the vicinity of 15 grams per 1,000 calories consumed. Here's the simple version:

The 2009–2010 National Health and Nutrition Examination Survey reported that the average caloric intake for Americans is just over 2,000 calories per day.

• According to the RAD eating plan, 2,000 calories equals 30 grams of fiber per day—the equivalent of two cups of cooked lentils, a cup of bran cereal, eight half-cup servings of collard greens, or eleven half-cup servings of broccoli.

• Also according to the RAD eating plan, 15% of 2,000 calories equals 300 calories from fat per day.

• Because fat contains 9 calories per gram, that equals 33 grams of fat per day—the equivalent of ten 3.5-ounce servings of skinless chicken, fourteen 3.5-ounce servings of broiled flounder, three eggs with the yolks included, or 2.5 ounces of almonds. Obviously, this is more chicken or fish than most people would eat in a day; the examples are provided to give you a sense of portion difference between fatty foods (eggs) and nonfatty foods (skinless chicken).

long-held belief that people with type 2 diabetes or prediabetes are best off eating a diet that restricts carbohydrate intake to half of their total calories is incorrect. In fact, a diet that's low in fat and high in carbohydrates—provided they are the right kind of carbs, such as vegetables, legumes, and whole grains—is not only beneficial, but appears to hold the key to improving insulin sensitivity, reducing body weight, and ultimately preventing or reversing type 2 diabetes.

The RAD Study Results: Better Insulin Sensitivity, Improved Glucose Control

One of the most remarkable results of our Rural Asian Diet Study was that our subjects showed significant improvements in insulin sensitivity and glucose control despite losing only a modest amount of weight—about 3% on average. In fact, a number of subjects recorded drops in their insulin levels on the diet despite not losing any weight—a clear indication that a high-fiber, low-fat diet improves insulin sensitivity and glucose control in ways that are *independent* of its weight-loss effects.

After eight weeks on the Rural Asian Diet . . .

- Both Asian Americans and Caucasian Americans experienced a 3% weight loss, on average, even when trying to *prevent* weight loss.

- Overall body fat and abdominal fat decreased in both groups.

- Both Asian Americans and Caucasian Americans had significantly reduced blood insulin levels—a sign of improved insulin sensitivity. Our Asian American subjects also recorded a significant drop in insulin resistance, as measured by the homeostatic model assessment method.

- Our Asian American study subjects also recorded a significant drop in blood glucose levels.

- In addition, all subjects showed a significant decrease in total cholesterol and LDL cholesterol levels after consuming the Rural Asian Diet.

Western Fast Food Isn't the Only Problem: How a *New York Times* Reporter Got the Story Wrong

When we talk about problematic modern diets, many people assume it's just Westernized food that's a problem. But as the rising diabetes epidemics in China, India, and other Asian countries illustrate, a Western-style high-fat diet can take hold virtually anywhere, simply by adding fat and removing fiber from the local cuisine. In China, rural regions still have very low diabetes rates, whereas the diabetes rate can be five times as high just one hundred miles away, in a more urbanized area.

Several years ago, *The New York Times* reported that fast food was causing the explosion of diabetes among Asian American populations in New York. Flushing, Queens, is a neighborhood that now has the largest Asian American population in New York City, more even than Chinatown in Manhattan. The diabetes rate in Flushing's Asian American community had skyrocketed in recent years, and the article's hypothesis was that this rise had occurred because the Asian community was flocking to fast-food restaurants such as McDonald's and KFC. There are close to a half million Asians living in Flushing while the area has only a relative handful of American fast-food restaurants, however, so it's hard to place all the blame on these establishments.

I believe that the main cause of diabetes in Flushing's Asian community was actually the *Asian* food the residents were consuming—which has changed totally in recent years. The rural food that first-generation Asian Americans grew up on contains very little oil and very little fat. It is generally steamed, not deep-fried, and the portions are much smaller than the portions served in Asian restaurants in Flushing and elsewhere in the United States.

Today, much of the Asian food served in urban areas has much more fat and is much higher in calories. Take one classic Chinese dish: beef and green pepper over rice and covered with sauce. Like many Asian dishes served in America, it has a very high oil content. In a part of New York with a concentration of Asian immigrants, this meal is sold for $4.00 and contains 1,200 calories—more than half a day's calories for many people.

There are plenty of other Asian menu items that are just as bad. If you want to write accurately about the epidemic of diabetes in this population, you have to address the issue of Westernized Asian food. There are many healthy Chinese dishes available as well. Thus, the key is to select those dishes that are tasty *and* healthy; this is not difficult. In addition, those Asian dishes that have been altered by a huge increase of fat or oil need to be reengineered to reduce their fat content.

Working the Fat Problem: Two Large-Scale Studies That Pointed the Way

I n developing the Rural Asian Diet, we've been guided largely by the historical eating patterns of populations that traditionally have had a very low incidence of type 2 diabetes. But the idea that reducing fat intake can prevent or reverse type 2 diabetes is also supported by two well-known multicenter, randomized controlled interventional studies. Although their targets for total fat intake aren't as low as ours, they were able to achieve some impressive results.

The Finnish Diabetes Prevention Study made history as one of the first randomized, controlled studies to show that type 2 diabetes can be prevented with lifestyle changes. The study, which took place from 1993 through 2000, followed 522 middle-aged, overweight subjects who had been diagnosed with impaired glucose tolerance, putting them at high risk of developing diabetes. They were randomly assigned to a "usual care" control group and to an intervention group that received individualized counseling aimed at cutting their daily fat intake to less than 30% of their total calories while getting at least 15 grams of fiber per 1,000 calories—the same fiber recommendation as the Rural Asian Diet. The intervention subjects were also encouraged to get at least thirty minutes of physical activity each day and were given the opportunity to receive resistance exercise training. When evaluated three years after starting their diabetes prevention protocol, subjects in the intervention group were 58% less likely to have developed type 2 diabetes than those in the control group. They had also maintained a weight loss of 7.5 pounds, compared to 2 pounds for the control group.

An even larger U.S. study, the Diabetes Prevention Program, followed more than 3,200 subjects who were overweight and had impaired glucose tolerance. The three-year study set a similar dietary target for its intervention group, encouraging them to reduce their daily fat intake to less than 30% of total calories while getting at least 150 minutes of physical activity per week. In this study, the intervention group was compared to a control group and a group that took the diabetes drug metformin. In addition to significant weight loss, which I'll describe in detail in the next chapter, the DPP intervention group showed an identical 58% reduction in their risk of getting type 2 diabetes compared to the control group. This was almost twice the risk reduction of the metformin group, which lowered their diabetes risk by 31%.

Putting the RAD Eating Plan into Action

I n this section, I'll explain how you can begin adapting the Rural Asian Diet to your own lifestyle. I'll start by sharing the basic principles of the RAD eating plan.

Principles of the Rural Asian Diet

- Base each meal on a creative mix of foods high in insoluble fiber, in the form of whole grains or pastas and vegetables.

- Add a moderate amount of animal protein to your plant base, preferably fish or shellfish. Remove poultry skin and trim away all visible fat from meat.

- If you aren't eating an animal protein, make sure that you eat a combination of legumes and whole grains to ensure that you're getting all the amino acids you need.

- Add fruit as desired.

- Strive for the "rainbow" effect by using as many different-colored vegetables, fruits, grains, and legumes as possible.

- Use only a moderate amount of monounsaturated oil (olive oil, canola oil, peanut oil, or safflower oil).

- Stick with low-calorie drinks such as water, tea, coffee, or vegetable juice (*not* fruit juice, which is high in sugar and low in fiber).

- Choose low-fat or nondairy alternatives.

- Avoid foods containing added sugar, high-fructose corn syrup and any foods containing partially hydrogenated vegetable oil (trans fats).

The Secret of the RAD Eating Plan: A Creative Mix of High-Fiber Foods

The two keys to the Rural Asian Diet are to keep fat intake low and eat a wide variety of foods that are high in plant-based fiber—enough so that you're consuming at least 15 grams for every 1,000 calories you eat. (The typical Western diet contains just 6 grams of fiber per 1,000 calories.) It's important to realize that there are two types of fiber contained in the plant foods you eat: *soluble* fiber (fiber that dissolves in water) and *insoluble* fiber (fiber that doesn't dissolve in water). Both types of fiber pass through the digestive system without being absorbed into the body, but they do this in different ways:

- Soluble fiber combines with water in your stomach and turns into a gel, which then tends to ferment in the colon. This gel slows the passage of digested food out of the stomach and through the intestine. Foods high in soluble fiber include oatmeal and oat bran, barley, nuts, seeds, beans, lentils, peas, some fruits (avocados, oranges, pears, bananas, blueberries, strawberries, prunes), and some vegetables (asparagus, Brussels sprouts, broccoli, carrots, celery, onions, sweet potatoes).

- Although insoluble fiber doesn't dissolve, it may absorb water and can also ferment in the intestinal tract, depending on which type it is. It tends to speed up the movement of food through the digestive tract. Insoluble fiber, particularly from whole grains, is the type of fiber *most closely associated with reduced risk of type 2 diabetes* in large-cohort population studies. Foods

Phasing in Fiber

If you're not accustomed to a high-fiber diet, transitioning to this kind of eating pattern too quickly can cause bloating and other gastrointestinal discomfort. For this reason, people used to low-fiber diets should gradually increase the amount of fiber they are eating over several weeks in order to reach the RAD target of 30 grams per day. Because dietary fiber absorbs water, you should also be sure to drink plenty of water and other fluids on a daily basis to avoid becoming dehydrated or constipated.

Whole Versus Processed Grains

There's a basic reason why whole grains are much better sources of dietary fiber than processed grains: When grains are processed, the whole point is to *remove* the harder, outer part of the grain—which is where the large majority of the fiber is, as well as the most of the grain's vitamins. Anytime a product label indicates that it is made simply with "wheat flour" (including "enriched," "bleached," or "unbleached" wheat flour), this means it's been made with kernels of grain but the fiber-rich husks have been removed. To be sure you're getting a whole grain in any store-bought food product you purchase, look for the word *whole* before the name of the grain, as in "whole wheat," "whole barley," or "whole rye." Whole-grain rice, on the other hand, will be listed as "brown rice." Note: Baked goods may contain a mix of whole wheat flour and (processed) wheat flour, both of which will then be listed on the label in order of the amount used. To be sure a product is made completely of whole grain, look for the "100% whole grain" stamp issued by the Whole Grains Council.

high in insoluble fiber include most vegetables, whole wheat and wheat bran, brown rice, and other whole grains.

THREE WORDS TO REMEMBER WHEN SHOPPING FOR VEGETABLES

Fresh, local, seasonal. Shop at farmer's markets whenever possible. If you don't have one nearby, join a local produce coop that provides and delivers fresh-grown vegetables. If you have access to neither, many grocery chains are partnering with local farmers to feature fresh produce. If the produce in your local store is not the best, fresh frozen vegetables are the next best thing—and often just as good in terms of nutritional value.

The Most Dangerous Fats

Although the Rural Asian Diet stresses reducing all fats, there are certain fats that are worse for your glucose metabolism than others. A variety of research indicates that two types of fat are strongly associated with increased risk of type 2 diabetes.

- **Saturated fats.** These fats are found primarily in meat; poultry skin; whole-fat dairy products including milk, cheese, and butter; and palm and coconut oil (which are common ingredients in commercial baked goods). These fats tend to be solid at room temperature because their chemical structures are "saturated" with hydrogen. Besides raising diabetes risk, eating saturated fats also boosts blood levels of dangerous LDL cholesterol and increases risk of cardiovascular disease.

- **Trans fats.** Most of these are artificially created fats, which are unsaturated fats (vegetable oils) that have been chemically treated to add additional hydrogen atoms to them. They are typically listed on food ingredient labels as "partially hydrogenated vegetable oil" or "vegetable shortening." Their chemical treatment makes them solid at room temperature instead of liquid, which makes them easier to transport and store, and less likely to spoil. Their chemical

RAD Low-Fat Substitution Tips

Unsure how to cut the fat out of your diet? Here are a number of simple ways to dramatically lower the fat content of some favorite food items.

HIGH FAT	LOW-FAT SUBSTITUTE
1 cup whole milk	1 cup skim milk
1 cup whipping cream	1 cup evaporated skim milk (chill well before whipping)
1 cup sour cream	1 cup low-fat or fat-free sour cream
1 ounce cream cheese	1 ounce light cream cheese
1 cup mayonnaise	1 cup light mayonnaise
1 whole egg	2 egg whites, or ¼ cup egg substitute
½ cup oil	½ cup applesauce (in baked goods)
1 tablespoon butter or margarine	1 tablespoon of a fat-free butter substitute*

* Butter substitutes that have 0 grams of fat include the following: I Can't Believe It's Not Butter Fat Free Spread; Promise Fat Free Spread; Smart Balance Buttery Burst Spray.

makeup also makes them very dangerous to your health: Trans fats not only elevate levels of dangerous LDL cholesterol but also lower levels of protective HDL cholesterol; they increase cardiovascular disease risk even more than saturated fats—which is why New York City and other localities have banned their use in restaurant food. In late 2013, the FDA proposed to remove trans fats from its "generally recognized as safe" category, which would be the first step toward banning these fats in the United States.

Because of diabetes and other health risks associated with saturated fats and trans fats, the Rural Asian Diet recommends avoiding trans fats completely and minimizing saturated fat intake by eating only meat that has had all visible fat removed, removing the skin from poultry before eating it, consuming only low-fat dairy products, and avoiding any baked goods containing palm and coconut oil. When using fats or oils to prepare meals or as a dressing for salads and other foods, select monounsaturated fats such as olive oil or canola oil, which appear to be significantly less harmful to glucose control and cardiovascular health.

Fifteen High-Fat Foods to Avoid

I f you're wondering what *not* to eat, here are fifteen foods that not only go into double digits in terms of the amount of fat grams you'll get per serving, but are also high in saturated fat.

FOOD (SERVING SIZE)	TOTAL FAT (GRAMS)
Bacon (3.5 oz)	50
Potato chips (3.5 oz)	35
Cheddar cheese (3.5 oz)	33
Corned beef (3.5 oz)	19
Ground beef (3.5 oz)	19
Bologna (regular beef 2 slices)	18
Chicken with skin (3.5 oz)	16
Ice cream (regular, 1 cup)	14
Hot dog (beef, 1)	14

FOOD (SERVING SIZE)	TOTAL FAT (GRAMS)
Croissant (1)	12
Doughnut (1)	12
Mayonnaise, regular (1 tablespoon)	11
Butter (1 tablespoon)	11
Steak (3.5 oz)	10
Cream cheese (regular, 1 oz)	10

Calculate Your Daily Fiber Intake

To estimate your average daily fiber intake, download this chart and print it out (you can find it at workman.com/thediabetesreset) or make a photocopy, and use the approximations listed in each category.

CEREALS	GRAMS OF FIBER PER SERVING	SERVINGS YOU EAT PER DAY	TOTAL GRAMS PER DAY
LOW-FIBER CEREALS Baked oat cereals, oatmeal, wheat flakes (½–¾ cup)	2–3		
MODERATE-FIBER CEREALS Bran flakes, shredded wheat, oat bran (½–¾ cup)	4–5		
HIGH-FIBER CEREALS Fiber One, All-Bran, 100% Bran, Bran Buds (⅓–½ cup)	8–12		
BREADS AND CRACKERS Whole-grain or whole wheat (1 serving/1 slice/1 ounce)	2–3		
GRAINS Couscous, bulgur, kasha, brown rice, barley (½ cup)	2–3		
STARCHY VEGETABLES Corn, peas (½ cup)	2–3		
VEGETABLES Cooked green beans, carrots, tomatoes, broccoli, etc. (½ cup)	2		
RAW VEGETABLES (1–2 cups)	3		

CEREALS	GRAMS OF FIBER PER SERVING	SERVINGS YOU EAT PER DAY	TOTAL GRAMS PER DAY
LEGUMES Dried peas, beans (black, red, kidney, pinto), lentils (⅓ cup)	4–5		
FRUITS ½ cup or 1 medium fresh fruit	2		
NUTS AND SEEDS ½ ounce	2		
FIBER SUPPLEMENT Check label			

The Rural Asian Diet Meal Planner

The RAD meal planner that follows includes a wide-ranging list of foods that can be eaten on the Rural Asian Diet, along with suggested guidelines on how to combine these foods into healthy meals that meet the RAD eating plan's targets of 70% carbohydrates, 15% fat, and 15% protein, with a minimum of 30 grams of fiber per day.

RAD FOOD LIST

A. Grains and Pasta

SERVING SIZE: ½ CUP (COOKED)	FIBER (GRAMS PER SERVING)	CALORIES PER SERVING
Brown rice	1.8	108
Bran cereal	14.2	60
Whole-grain corn pasta	3.4	88
Whole-grain wheat pasta and noodles	3.2	87
Soba noodles	0.0	56
Quinoa	2.6	111
Brown rice pilaf	1.5	105
Farro	4.0	100
Kamut	3.7	114
Kasha	2.3	77

SERVING SIZE: ½ CUP (COOKED)	FIBER (GRAMS PER SERVING)	CALORIES PER SERVING
Wild rice	1.5	83
Whole wheat couscous	1.1	88
Oatmeal	2.0	75
Whole wheat bread (1 slice)	1.9	81
Whole wheat English muffin (1 muffin)	4.4	134

B. Starchy Vegetables

SERVING SIZE: ½ CUP (COOKED)	FIBER (GRAMS PER SERVING)	CALORIES PER SERVING
Sweet potatoes	3.3	90
Pumpkin	1.3	24
Winter squash	2.9	38
Sweet corn (½ large ear)	1.4	62
Peas	2.2	34
Parsnip	2.8	55
Rutabaga	1.5	26
Water chestnuts	1.9	60
Chestnuts	0.0	22
Taro	3.4	94

C. Nonstarchy Vegetables

SERVING SIZE: ½ CUP	FIBER (GRAMS PER SERVING)	CALORIES PER SERVING
Spinach (cooked)	2.2	21
Lettuce (green, raw)	0.2	3
Bell peppers (raw)	1.3	15
Tomato (raw)	0.7	13
Carrots (raw)	1.8	26
Asparagus (cooked)	1.8	20

SERVING SIZE: ½ CUP	FIBER (GRAMS PER SERVING)	CALORIES PER SERVING
Mushroom (cooked)	1.0	14
Onion (yellow, sautéed)	0.7	57
Broccoli (cooked)	2.6	27
Cucumber (peeled, raw)	0.5	8
Eggplant (cooked)	1.2	17
Kale (cooked)	1.3	18
Green beans (cooked)	4.0	44
Baked beans (canned vegetarian)	5.2	119
Collard greens (cooked)	3.8	31
Brussels sprouts (cooked)	2.0	28
Celery (raw)	0.8	8
Alfalfa sprouts (raw)	0.3	4
Sprouted mung beans (raw)	0.9	16
Cauliflower (raw)	1.1	13
Cauliflower (cooked)	1.4	14
Summer squash (cooked)	1.0	17

Why Slow Eating and Moderate Portions Are Essential If You Have Diabetes

Where glucose metabolism is concerned, being careful not to eat too fast or too much in one sitting is also important. I recommend that anyone with prediabetes or diabetes avoid eating overly large meals and chew each mouthful of food at least ten times before swallowing it. Here's why: If you have diabetes and you eat too quickly, or eat a large amount of food or a high-fat meal, this can frequently cause your glucose levels to reach a higher peak than usual following your meal. This is due to several factors, including nerve dysfunction in the intestines, which some diabetic patients suffer from, that prevents their digestive system from handling large volumes of food effectively. In addition, many people with diabetes don't have a sufficient insulin reserve to control their glucose levels if they take in food too quickly.

D. Legumes

SERVING SIZE: ¼ CUP (COOKED)	FIBER (GRAMS PER SERVING)	CALORIES PER SERVING
Lentils	7.8	115
Soy beans/edamame	3.8	127
Kidney beans	6.5	112
Black beans	7.5	114
Chickpeas	6.2	134
Lima beans	6.6	108
Fava beans	4.6	94
Hummus	7.4	204
Natto	4.7	186

E. Fruits

SERVING SIZE: ½ CUP (RAW)	FIBER (GRAMS PER SERVING)	CALORIES PER SERVING
Orange	2.2	43
Grapefruit	1.3	34
Strawberries	1.5	24
Raspberries	4.0	32
Apple (with skin)	1.5	32
Banana	2.0	67
Blueberries	1.8	42
Pear	2.2	40
Peach	1.2	30
Cantaloupe	0.8	30
Lemon (without peel)	3.0	31
Grapes	0.4	31
Raisins	3.1	247

F. Protein

SERVING SIZE: 100 G/3.5 OZ	FAT (GRAMS PER SERVING)	CALORIES PER SERVING
Tofu (silken, firm)	2.7	62
Part-skim mozzarella cheese	20.0	302
Low-fat cottage cheese (1% fat)	1.0	72
Salmon	8.0	182
Sardines (canned in oil)	11.5	208
Mackerel	17.0	262
Tuna (broiled)	6.0	184
Tuna (canned in water)	3.0	128
Bluefish	5.5	159
Cod	0.9	105
Tilapia	2.7	128
Flounder	2.4	86
Halibut	1.6	111
Skinless chicken (braised)	3.2	157
Skinless turkey	2.0	130
Lean pork	3.5	143
Lean beef	8.5	183
Egg	10.6	155
Egg white	0.2	52

G. Nuts and Seeds

SERVING SIZE: 1 OZ	FAT (GRAMS PER SERVING)	FIBER (GRAMS PER SERVING)	CALORIES PER SERVING
Almonds	14.0	3.5	164
Walnuts	18.5	1.9	185
Sunflower seeds	14.6	2.4	166
Pumpkin seeds	13.9	1.7	158
Cashews	12.4	0.9	157

SERVING SIZE: 1 OZ	FAT (GRAMS PER SERVING)	FIBER (GRAMS PER SERVING)	CALORIES PER SERVING
Pecans	20.0	2.7	196
Pistachios	12.9	2.9	159
Peanuts	14.0	2.4	161

Processed (and Red) Meat: Just Say "No"

If you have prediabetes or type 2 diabetes and you're thinking of getting bacon or sausage with your breakfast or grabbing a hot dog at the ball game, think twice: In a study published in 2011 by our colleagues at the Harvard University School of Public Health, they combined data from a number of long-term studies encompassing nearly a half million people and found that those who ate a daily serving of just *50 grams of processed meat*—the amount found in one hot dog or sausage, or two slices of bacon—had a 51% increased risk of developing type 2 diabetes compared to the population as a whole. The study also found that a daily *100-gram serving of nonprocessed red meat* increased type 2 diabetes risk by 19%.

The researchers conjectured that the extra high risk associated with processed meat may be related to their high content of nitrites and nitrates, which are used to preserve the meat. These compounds are converted by the digestive system into related compounds called nitrosamines, which are toxic to the beta cells of the pancreas and can also impair the body's response to insulin. The researchers also noted that red meat consumption is associated with increased systemic inflammation and weight gain, and that the iron in red meat can also promote the production of free radicals, contributing to oxidative stress.

H. Fats

SERVING SIZE: 1 TABLESPOON	FAT (GRAMS PER SERVING)	CALORIES PER SERVING
Olive oil	13.5	119
Canola oil	14.0	124
Grapeseed oil	13.6	120

SERVING SIZE: 1 TABLESPOON	FAT (GRAMS PER SERVING)	CALORIES PER SERVING
Peanut oil	13.5	119
Safflower oil	13.6	120
Sesame oil	13.6	120
Avocado (1 oz)	2.6	50
Olives (1 oz)	4.3	41

I. Dairy and Dairy Alternatives

SERVING SIZE: 1 CUP (8 OZ)	FAT (GRAMS PER SERVING)	CALORIES PER SERVING
Low-fat yogurt (plain)	3.5	143
1% milk	2.4	105
Fat-free milk	0.6	91
Unsweetened soy milk	4.0	80
Unsweetened almond milk	3.5	40
Unsweetened rice milk	2.0	45

J. Condiments, Pastes, Spreads, and Dips

SERVING SIZE: 1 TABLESPOON	FAT (GRAMS PER SERVING)	CALORIES PER SERVING
Low-fat mayonnaise	4.0	45
Low-sodium miso	1.0	34
Mustard (Dijon)	0.0	5
Worcestershire sauce	0.0	13
Pickle relish (sweet)	0.07	20
Soy sauce (low sodium)	0.05	14
Teriyaki sauce	0.0	16
Soynut butter	13.6	120
Almond butter	8.9	98
Tapenade	4.0	40

SERVING SIZE: 1 TABLESPOON	FAT (GRAMS PER SERVING)	CALORIES PER SERVING
Baba ghanoush	1.9	24
Fat-free butter substitutes	0.0	5

K. Beverages

SERVING SIZE: 1 CUP (8 OZ)	FIBER (GRAMS PER SERVING)	CALORIES PER SERVING
Water	0.0	0
Tea	0.0	2
Coffee	0.0	2
Aojiru juice	1.0	63
Carrot juice	1.9	94
Low-sodium tomato juice	1.0	41

L. Herbs and Spices

Ginger	Parsley	Peppermint	Sage
Basil	Lemon balm	Tarragon	Rosemary

Rural Asian Diet Meal Plans

U se these meal plans as outlines for creating your own individualized meals, drawing from the food list starting on page 56.

- Always use the 2–1–1 formula for whatever meal you're eating: two portions of nonstarchy vegetables; one portion of whole grains, legumes, or starchy vegetables; and one portion of protein, with a piece of fruit on the side.

- Avoid canned foods, which tend to be high in sodium, and commercial baked goods other than whole-grain breads and crackers.

- Frozen vegetables are fine, as long as there are no added ingredients.

- When cooking with oils or using oils in dressings, choose only the oils on the RAD food list, and use as sparingly as possible.

- Be moderate in your consumption of all low-fat dairy products (which still contain some fat, unless they are fat-free or made from skim milk) as well as nuts (which can also be surprisingly high in fat), and try to keep track of how many grams of fats you consume from these sources.

- Always choose broth-based soups and avoid all cream-based soups, dressings, and sauces.

- When eating out, choose foods that have been grilled, steamed, poached, or baked rather than fried or sautéed.

Mixing and Matching the RAD Meal Plans

E ach individual meal plan listed follows the low-fat, high-fiber guidelines of the RAD eating plan. To plan your menus for the day or the week, simply combine these suggested breakfast, lunch, and dinner menus in any way you like. Because my eating plan calls for restricting calories *only* if you are engaged in a period of targeted weight loss, other readers can generally select their own individual portion sizes, provided these portions give you enough dietary fiber and don't contain more fat, in total, than your daily limit for fat grams (from meats, poultry, dairy products, nuts, and foods made with oils). The overall amount of food you eat at each meal should not be excessive, however, because an overly large meal (or one eaten too quickly) will produce an excessive insulin response after eating. In general, following the portion sizes outlined in the RAD food list is a good starting point.

If you are going through a period of targeted weight loss, then you should begin by analyzing the calories contained in the portion sizes listed in the RAD food list: 3.5 ounces for meat and poultry; ½ cup for vegetables, grains, legumes, fruit, and dairy products; 1 ounce for nuts; and 1 tablespoon for oils. From there, you can modify these serving sizes as needed in order to stay within your daily calorie limits.

RAD Breakfast Plans

EGGS

Egg omelet with vegetables

Egg-white frittata with vegetables

Egg substitute scrambled eggs with vegetables

PANCAKES

Whole-grain pancakes

GRAINS

Oatmeal with low-fat yogurt

Bran cereal with low-fat milk

Whole-grain toast or English muffin with nut butter

YOGURT OR SMOOTHIE

Low-fat Greek yogurt with fruit added

Smoothie (soy milk, almond milk, or rice milk with fruit add-ons)

Add-ons to previous meals. Fruit (banana, cantaloupe, grapefruit, orange, apple), nuts, vegetable juice, coffee, or tea

ASIAN-STYLE

Brown rice with miso soup, teriyaki chicken, or tofu stew

Tofu wakame udon (tofu, scallions, noodles and broth, wakame)

Add-ons. Soy milk, grapes, oranges, apples, brown rice congee, aojiru juice

RAD Lunch Plans

THE PERFECT PLATE (BASED ON A STANDARD 9-INCH PLATE)

One-fourth plate contains cooked whole grains, legumes, or starchy vegetables; one-half plate contains nonstarchy vegetables (steamed, boiled, or sautéed); one-fourth plate contains lean fish, poultry, or meat (baked, grilled, pan-broiled, or broiled). Vegetarian alternative: add eggs, cheese, or legumes to replace protein portion.

SALADS
Green salad with low-fat dressing
Vegetable salad with grain and protein add-ons
Whole-grain or bean salad
Grilled chicken salad (made with low-fat mayonnaise) with fruit and
　　vegetable add-ons
Tuna chunk salad (low-fat mayo) with fruit and vegetable add-ons

SOUPS
Low-sodium vegetable, chicken, or bean soup

SANDWICHES
Whole-grain bread, low-fat condiments, greens, sprouts, tomato, avocado,
　　with: low-fat cheese, low-fat chicken salad, or low-fat tuna salad

GRAINS, PASTA, OR PIZZA
Cooked whole grains with vegetable, meat, poultry, or seafood add-ons
Whole-grain pasta with vegetable, meat, poultry, or seafood add-ons
Whole-grain pizza with vegetable and low-fat cheese add-ons

GRILLED
Shish kabob (cubes of protein food and assorted vegetables)
Grilled meat, chicken, or fish and/or vegetables

YOGURT-SMOOTHIE
Yogurt with fruit added
Smoothie (soy milk, almond milk, or rice milk with fruit add-ons)

Add-ons to previous meals. Raw vegetables (with dip if desired), vegetable
　　juice, whole-grain bread, fruit (banana, cantaloupe, apple, grapes), nuts
　　and seeds, low-fat cheese, hummus, baba ghanoush, tapenade

ASIAN-STYLE
Pork, chicken, or tofu with vegetables over brown rice or noodles
Fried rice with vegetables and shrimp, pork, or chicken
Stir-fry vegetable, meat, or poultry dishes over brown rice or noodles
Add-ons. Soup, fruit (apple, grapes, pear, orange), vegetable juice

RAD Dinner Plans

THE PERFECT PLATE (BASED ON A STANDARD 9-INCH PLATE)

One-fourth plate contains cooked whole grains, legumes, or starchy vegetables; one-half plate contains nonstarchy vegetables (steamed, boiled, or sautéed); one-fourth plate contains lean fish, poultry, or meat (baked, grilled, pan-broiled, or broiled). Vegetarian alternative: add eggs, cheese, or legumes to replace protein portion.

GRILLED

Shish kabob (cubes of protein food and assorted vegetables)

Grilled meat, chicken, or fish

Grilled vegetables

GRAINS OR PASTA

Cooked whole grains with vegetable, meat, poultry, or seafood add-ons

Whole-grain pasta with vegetable, meat, poultry, or seafood add-ons

SALAD

Vegetable salad with cooked grains and protein add-ons

Grain or bean salad

Chicken or tuna salad (made with low-fat mayonnaise) with fruit, nut, or
   vegetable add-ons

SOUPS

Low-sodium vegetable, chicken, or bean soup

Add-ons to previous meals. Raw vegetables (with dip if desired), salad
   with low-fat dressing, whole-grain bread, fruit (banana, cantaloupe,
   apple, grapes), nuts or seeds, low-fat cheese, hummus, baba ghanoush,
   tapanade

ASIAN-STYLE

Pork, chicken, or tofu with vegetables over brown rice or noodles

Fried rice with vegetables and shrimp, pork, or chicken

Stir-fry vegetable, meat, or poultry dishes over brown rice or noodles

Add-ons. Soup, fruit (apple, grapes, pear, orange), vegetable juice

RAD Snack Suggestions

VERY LOW-CARB

Fresh vegetable juice or low-sodium vegetable juice

Boiled string beans and carrots wrapped in low-sodium seaweed

Sliced cucumber with miso dip (1 tablespoon low-sodium miso and
½ tablespoon vinegar)

Mixed vegetable soup

Steamed egg in low-sodium broth or water (you can add mushrooms,
scallions, or ginger)

Hard-boiled egg

Vegetable salad

LOW CARBOHYDRATE (LESS THAN 10 GRAMS OF CARBS PER SERVING)

Edamame, boiled or steamed

Unsweetened soy milk or almond milk

Almond milk

Tofu pudding

Nuts

Whole-grain bread with nut butter or low-fat cheese

Sliced bell peppers with dip (try imitation crab meat: 2 ounces with
2 teaspoons light mayo and cilantro)

MODERATE CARBOHYDRATE (LESS THAN 20 GRAMS OF CARBS PER SERVING)

Fruit

Hummus with celery and carrots

Applesauce (no sugar added)

Yogurt

Sugar-free pudding

Sugar-free hot chocolate

Whole-grain crackers

Hard-boiled egg or scrambled egg on whole wheat toast

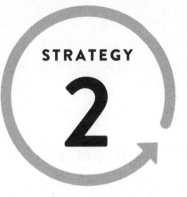

2

REDUCE YOUR BODY WEIGHT BY 5% TO 7%

Excess body fat interferes with insulin sensitivity through several different mechanisms. If your BMI is above 25 and you are able to reduce your body weight by 5% to 7%, you can reduce your insulin resistance and improve your glucose metabolism significantly. This chapter explains why losing a relatively modest amount of weight is so important in diabetes prevention, and the best way to accomplish this.

I f you've been diagnosed with prediabetes or type 2 diabetes or have been warned you may have prediabetes or signs of insulin resistance, in addition to adopting the Rural Asian Diet, there is another thing you can start doing *today* that will significantly improve your condition in just a few weeks: The evidence is clear that reducing your body weight by 5% or more is the *single most effective step* you can take to immediately begin increasing your insulin sensitivity and start reversing your type 2 diabetes or prediabetes.

Even just a couple of pounds of weight loss is likely to cause some improvement in your body's insulin sensitivity and your ability to metabolize blood glucose. If you're able to go further, and follow a targeted weight-loss program that lowers your body weight by at least 5% (10 pounds, for someone weighing 200 pounds), you will see a significant improvement in your blood glucose control and will also significantly reduce your risk of developing diabetes and all of the complications related to it.

Studying the Obesity-Diabetes Link

Although doctors have known for many years that being overweight—or, more accurately, overfat—seems to be associated with a higher prevalence of type 2 diabetes, we've only recently been able to pin down the statistical relationship and, even more important, start to understand the mechanisms underlying this connection. Over the past twenty years, a number of research projects have studied large groups of people in an attempt to determine exactly how being overweight affects your risk of developing insulin resistance or type 2 diabetes. As a result of these studies, the link between excess body fat and impaired glucose control is now clear. In 2009, a team of Canadian researchers published a meta-analysis (a study that analyzes the results of many previous research projects) of eighty-nine studies on the relationship between obesity and various medical conditions. The meta-analysis (which analyzes the combined results of multiple studies by other labs) concluded that men who are obese—meaning that their BMI is 30 or higher—are seven times more likely to develop diabetes than men with "normal" BMIs, under 25. The same analysis also found that women with a BMI of 30 or above were even more at risk, being twelve times more likely to get diabetes than normal-weight women.

For people who are extremely obese, with a BMI of 35 or above, the diabetes risk is even greater: Studies have found that men and women in this category are about forty times more likely to develop type 2 diabetes than lean individuals. Just as striking, when they are able to lower their BMI to a normal level, most people with diabetes see significant improvements in their condition. Often they can be weaned off diabetes medication completely and maintain good glucose control on a monitored program of diet and exercise.

What's Your BMI, and Why Does It Matter?

Your BMI is calculated by taking your mass in kilograms and then dividing it by your height in meters squared (the number you get by multiplying your height in meters times itself). If, like most Americans, you're accustomed to measuring your height and weight in inches and pounds, then you can get your BMI by taking your weight in pounds, dividing it by your height in inches squared, then multiplying the total by 703. Using this method, the BMI for someone who weighs 200 pounds and is six feet (72 inches) tall, would be calculated as follows:

$(200 / (72)^2) \times 703 = (200 / 5184) \times 703 = .0386 \times 703 = 27.1$

Use the chart on page 72 to find your BMI.

A BMI below 25 is generally considered normal weight, whereas someone with a BMI of 25 to 30 is considered to be officially overweight. A BMI of 30 to 35 puts you in the "obese" category, and a BMI of 35 or greater is considered "extremely obese." For Asians and Asian Americans, these cutoff points are lower—24 to 27 is considered overweight, and 27 or above is considered obese.

Waist Circumference—Another Way of Measuring Dangerous Abdominal Fat

While these BMI categories are useful up to a point, many doctors and scientists feel that BMI is actually of limited value in determining a person's risk for prediabetes and diabetes because it doesn't distinguish between the amount of fat and lean tissue that person is carrying on their body. As we get older, we tend to lose muscle mass and gain fat, putting us at increased risk of diabetes even if our weight stays the same. BMI also doesn't make a distinction between different types of body fat. Because abdominal fat is the most dangerous type of fat in terms of diabetes risk, many doctors use people's *waist circumference* as an additional measurement to estimate abdominal fat content.

	90LB 40.9 KG	95LB 43.2 KG	100LB 45.5 KG	105LB 47.7 KG	110LB 50.0 KG	115LB 52.3 KG	120LB 54.5 KG	125LB 56.8 KG	130LB 59.1 KG	135LB 61.4 KG	140LB 63.6 KG	145LB 65.9 KG	150LB 68.2 KG
4'10" 147 CM	18.8	19.9	20.9	22.0	23.0	24.1	25.1	26.2	27.2	28.3	29.3	30.4	31
4'11" 150 CM	18.2	19.2	20.2	21.3	22.3	23.3	24.3	25.3	26.3	27.3	28.3	29.3	30
5'0" 152 CM	17.6	18.6	19.6	20.5	21.5	22.5	23.5	24.5	25.4	26.4	27.4	28.4	29
5'1" 155 CM	17.0	18.0	18.9	19.9	20.8	21.8	22.7	23.7	24.6	25.6	26.5	27.5	28
5'2" 157 CM	16.5	17.4	18.3	19.2	20.2	21.1	22.0	22.9	23.8	24.7	25.7	26.6	27
5'3" 160 CM	16.0	16.9	17.8	18.6	19.5	20.4	21.3	22.2	23.1	24.0	24.9	25.7	26
5'4" 163 CM	15.5	16.3	17.2	18.1	18.9	19.8	20.6	21.5	22.4	23.2	24.1	24.9	25
5'5" 165 CM	15.0	15.8	16.7	17.5	18.3	19.2	20.0	20.8	21.7	22.5	23.3	24.2	25
5'6" 168 CM	14.6	15.4	16.2	17.0	17.8	18.6	19.4	20.2	21.0	21.8	22.6	23.5	24
5'7" 170 CM	14.1	14.9	15.7	16.5	17.3	18.0	18.8	19.6	20.4	21.2	22.0	22.8	2
5'8" 173 CM	13.7	14.5	15.2	16.0	16.8	17.5	18.3	19.0	19.8	20.6	21.3	22.1	2
5'9" 175 CM	13.3	14.1	14.8	15.5	16.3	17.0	17.8	18.5	19.2	20.0	20.7	21.5	2
5'10" 178 CM	12.9	13.7	14.4	15.1	15.8	16.5	17.3	18.0	18.7	19.4	20.1	20.8	2
5'11" 180 CM	12.6	13.3	14.0	14.7	15.4	16.1	16.8	17.5	18.2	18.9	19.6	20.3	2
6'0" 183 CM	12.2	12.9	13.6	14.3	14.9	15.6	16.3	17.0	17.7	18.3	19.0	19.7	20
6'1" 185 CM	11.9	12.6	13.2	13.9	14.5	15.2	15.9	16.5	17.2	17.8	18.5	19.2	19
6'2" 188 CM	11.6	12.2	12.9	13.5	14.2	14.8	15.4	16.1	16.7	17.4	18.0	18.7	19

For most ethnic groups, a BMI of 25 or above means you are overweight, and a BMI of 30 or above means you are obese.
For individuals of Asian descent, a BMI of 24 or above is considered overweight, and a BMI of 27 or above is considered obese.

| B | 160LB | 165LB | 170LB | 175LB | 180LB | 185LB | 190LB | 195LB | 200LB | 205LB | 210LB | 215LB | 220LB |
KG	72.7 KG	75.0 KG	77.3 KG	79.5 KG	81.8 KG	84.1 KG	86.4 KG	88.6 KG	90.9 KG	93.2 KG	95.5 KG	97.7 KG	100 KG
	33.5	34.6	35.6	36.7	37.7	38.7	39.8	40.8	41.9	42.9	44.0	45.0	46.1
	32.4	33.4	34.4	35.4	36.4	37.4	38.5	39.5	40.5	41.5	42.5	43.5	44.5
	31.3	32.3	33.3	34.2	35.2	36.2	37.2	38.2	39.1	40.1	41.1	42.1	43.1
	30.3	31.2	32.2	33.1	34.1	35.0	36.0	36.9	37.9	38.8	39.8	40.7	41.7
	29.3	30.2	31.2	32.1	33.0	33.9	34.8	35.7	36.7	37.6	38.5	39.4	40.3
	28.4	29.3	30.2	31.1	32.0	32.8	33.7	34.6	35.5	36.4	37.3	38.2	39.1
	27.5	28.4	29.2	30.1	31.0	31.8	32.7	33.5	34.4	35.3	36.1	37.0	37.8
	26.7	27.5	28.3	29.2	30.0	30.8	31.7	32.5	33.4	34.2	35.0	35.9	36.7
	25.9	26.7	27.5	28.3	29.1	29.9	30.7	31.5	32.3	33.2	34.0	34.8	35.6
	25.1	25.9	26.7	27.5	28.3	29.0	29.8	30.6	31.4	32.2	33.0	33.7	34.5
	24.4	25.1	25.9	26.7	27.4	28.2	28.9	29.7	30.5	31.2	32.0	32.8	33.5
	23.7	24.4	25.2	25.9	26.6	27.4	28.1	28.9	29.6	30.3	31.1	31.8	32.6
	23.0	23.7	24.4	25.2	25.9	26.6	27.3	28.0	28.8	29.5	30.2	30.9	31.6
	22.4	23.1	23.8	24.5	25.2	25.9	26.6	27.3	28.0	28.7	29.4	30.0	30.7
	21.7	22.4	23.1	23.8	24.5	25.1	25.8	26.5	27.2	27.9	28.5	29.2	29.9
	21.2	21.8	22.5	23.1	23.8	24.5	25.1	25.8	26.4	27.1	27.8	28.4	29.1
	20.6	21.2	21.9	22.5	23.2	23.8	24.4	25.1	25.7	26.4	27.0	27.7	28.3

To measure your waist circumference, run a tape measure completely around your abdomen, level with the top of your hip bones and even with your belly button or just above it. Make sure that the tape is horizontal and pressed snugly against your skin, but not so snug that it makes an indentation.

WHAT THE RESULTS MEAN:
For men with a BMI of 25 or above, a waist circumference greater than 40 inches is considered an indication of significant abdominal fat deposits and high risk for type 2 diabetes. For women with a BMI in that range, a waist circumference of more than 35 inches is an indicator of high diabetes risk. Any increase in waist circumference over time is also a cause for concern as well because this is a sign that you are accumulating abdominal fat.

All of these measurements have their place, and you may want to talk to your doctor about keeping track of your own BMI and waist circumference. If you have diabetes or prediabetes, however, the most important statistics are *what you weigh now and how much weight you're able to lose* in the coming weeks and months. As I'll explain in this chapter, every pound you shed reduces the size of your fat cells and the total amount of fat you're storing in your body, both of which lead to improvements in your body's ability to utilize insulin and metabolize the glucose in your bloodstream.

Not Everyone Who Weighs Too Much Has Type 2 Diabetes, but Almost Everyone with Type 2 Diabetes Weighs Too Much

It's important to realize that although obesity is a leading risk factor for type 2 diabetes, this does *not* mean that everyone who weighs too much is destined to develop diabetes. The latest surveys show that 36% of American adults—slightly more than one third—are obese, and another 33% are overweight (meaning their BMI is between 25 and 30),

The Link Between Expanding Fat Cells
and Insulin Resistance

The average adult has about 30 billion fat cells in his or her body. When people gain additional body fat, these cells begin to increase their size (hypertrophy) in order to hold the added fat, which is stored as triglyceride droplets. A fat cell can expand to about four times its normal size, at which point it can no longer hold any more fat. If someone continues to gain weight beyond this point, the body will begin creating new fat cells. As you'll see in this chapter, the underlying mechanisms of insulin resistance are related in large part to the chemical changes that occur as fat cells grow larger—including the fact that this hypertrophy leads to an increased flux of fatty acids out of the fat stores and also stimulates fat cells to produce inflammatory cytokines (immune system proteins that trigger an inflammatory response on body tissue).

or obese. Yet only between 8% and 9% of the adult population in the United States has type 2 diabetes.

If you drill down into the statistics about who does and doesn't develop diabetes, it becomes clear that, like so many other diabetes risk factors, the obesity-diabetes link involves the combination of an innate vulnerability meeting a precipitating trigger. If someone with no family history of diabetes is overweight or obese, she has less than a 10% chance of becoming diabetic despite the excess fat she is carrying. Studies suggest that one reason for this somewhat protective effect may be due to the fact that this "nonfamily history" group is less prone to develop the inflammatory response that excess body weight is often associated with—a phenomenon I discuss in more detail.

It should also be pointed out that a minority of those people who have type 2 diabetes—about 20%—are *not* overweight or obese. In addition, a fair number of lean individuals, particularly those with two parents who were diagnosed with type 2 diabetes, show signs of insulin resistance early in adulthood. These are clear indications that factors other than excess body fat, including some inherited characteristics, are contributing to at least some cases of prediabetes and diabetes.

That said, it's also clear that for most people with diabetes or pre-diabetes, excess body fat is playing a significant role in their condition. As noted previously, among those American adults who *do* have type 2 diabetes, 80% are overweight or obese. The diabetes risk associated with being overfat is even greater if you have a genetic vulnerability: If you have two parents with type 2 diabetes and you are merely overweight, which means simply having a BMI over 25, you have an *80% chance* of eventually developing diabetes.

These statistics suggest that if you do have type 2 diabetes or pre-diabetes, or even if you're just showing early signs of insulin resistance, excess body fat is almost certainly contributing to your condition to some extent—which also implies that shedding some of that fat will help improve your ability to metabolize blood glucose.

Debunking the Media: Why "Eating Less and Moving More" Is Not Only Good Advice, but the Only Tested and Proven Advice

MEDIA MYTH: BECAUSE YOUR METABOLISM SLOWS WHEN YOU CUT CALORIE INTAKE, IT IS ALMOST IMPOSSIBLE TO LOSE WEIGHT.

This myth was recently put forward by one self-styled weight-loss expert, who claimed that because our metabolisms slow and our appetites increase when we cut our daily caloric intake—the "set point" concept—the advice that people should eat less and exercise more in order to lose weight constitutes part of the "lie" that losing weight is a matter of willpower.

It is certainly true that people's metabolisms will tend to slow down as they restrict their caloric intake. This is known as the "set point" effect, in which the body tries to preserve its weight at its existing (over-weight) level. Experts widely agree that the set point phenomenon poses a major challenge to successful weight loss. But as you'll see in this chapter, the conclusion that calorie restriction plus exercise is therefore a useless formula flies in the face of numerous large-scale weight-loss studies, including the clinical results of Joslin's weight-loss program—all of which show that many of thousands of people have been able to achieve significant weight loss by restricting their calories for a limited amount of time while increasing their daily physical activity.

The set point usually manifests itself through an increase in appetite that can be very powerful. The RAD eating plan's recommendations to eat foods that are high in fiber and good tasting are designed to neutralize this aspect of the set point by providing maximum feelings of satiety for the amount of calories you consume.

It's also clear that people's set points can be changed, as demonstrated by the fact that people are able to dramatically decrease the amount of food they take in following bariatric surgery or as the result of treatment with medications such as incretins (also called GLP-1 agonists). In addition, Europeans tend to be much thinner than European Americans with a similar genetic background. If the set point for weight is really so all-controlling, then it must be genetically determined—but if that is true, then it becomes very hard to explain the clear BMI difference between inhabitants of the two continents.

This conclusion also ignores the fact that daily exercise, far from being useless, is actually the single most effective way to counter the set point–related metabolic slowdown associated with eating in a healthier way and consuming fewer calories. In fact, altering one's energy balance by taking in fewer calories per day while making an effort to expend calories through daily physical activity is not only an effective way to lose weight, but it's the *only* approach that has consistently been proven by large-scale clinical trials to help people reduce their weight without surgery or medications.

MEDIA MYTH: BECAUSE THERE IS SO MUCH "CONFLICTING ADVICE" ABOUT HOW TO LOSE WEIGHT, IT'S IMPOSSIBLE TO KNOW HOW TO PROCEED WITH CONFIDENCE.

First of all, a major reason why there are so many different weight-loss approaches presented in the media is simply that weight loss sells. Books offering various diets are a staple on the bestseller lists, and a cover article on the latest silver bullet for losing weight is certain to boost newsstand sales of any magazine. Another reason why there are a multitude of different diet plans is that virtually any eating strategy that cuts your total calories will be effective for losing weight—including low-fat, high-fiber approaches like my RAD eating plan, as well as low-carb, high-fat strategies like the Atkins and high-protein diets. I endorse a low-fat, high-fiber diet because it's not only effective for losing weight, but it also maximizes the function of your glucose metabolism and is by far the healthiest way to eat over a lifetime.

That said, I encourage anyone who needs to lose weight in order to improve their glucose metabolism to find an approach that works for you. And again, far from being "conflicting," all of the truly effective weight-loss strategies out there boil down to the same thing: Cut your daily calorie intake for several months, through whatever combination of healthy foods works best for you, while getting thirty minutes or more of exercise most days of the week.

How Does Excess Body Fat Cause Diabetes?

Although the statistical link between excess body fat and impaired ability to metabolize blood glucose has been evident for quite some time, the biological mechanisms underlying this link remained elusive until recently. Over the past decade, however, researchers at Joslin and elsewhere have identified a number of ways that the body's ability to metabolize glucose becomes disrupted as people gain excess weight:

EXCESS BODY FAT LEADS TO FAT DEPOSITS INSIDE YOUR MUSCLE CELLS THAT INTERFERE WITH INSULIN SIGNALING.

One source of insulin resistance appears to be tiny deposits of fat inside the muscle cells, which have been shown to interfere with the ability of insulin to transport glucose into the muscles. As I discuss in detail in Strategy Chapter 3, your skeletal muscles—the muscles that you use constantly to move your arms, legs, head, and other body parts—are the tissues that are primarily responsible for metabolizing the "insulin-mediated" glucose in your bloodstream. (Your brain also uses a great deal of glucose, but doesn't require insulin to metabolize it.) Insulin resistance (loss of insulin sensitivity) in the skeletal muscles is now considered to be one of the primary causes of type 2 diabetes.

These fat deposits accumulate in your muscles' cells as the result of several factors. One is an increase in flux of fatty acids from the body's fat stores (the large fat deposits in your body) into the body's peripheral tissues, including muscle tissue. This increased flux happens as a person's body fat content—especially abdominal fat—rises. One reason for this is that as the body's fat stores become greater, there tends to be more "spillover" of fats into other parts of the body. Another reason is that as a person becomes fatter and more insulin resistant, this insulin resistance creates a vicious cycle by increasing the tendency of the body to metabolize its fat stores and send fatty acids out through the bloodstream to other parts of the body.

Although this increase in the flux of fatty acids doesn't reduce your fat stores (because you're still storing fat at the same time), it does increase the amount of circulating fatty acids that can be taken up by the muscles. For many people, another important contributing factor is an impaired ability of the muscles to burn (oxidize) fatty acids for fuel. Although muscles use glucose for fuel during times of high activity, they also use fatty acids for fuel, especially in times of lower activity. If they aren't burning this fat efficiently, fats start to accumulate inside the muscles' cells instead.

This impaired fat-burning ability is often due at least in part to lack of fitness as a result of physical inactivity. For a number of people with prediabetes or diabetes, it's also due partly to inherited deficiencies in the muscles' mitochondria (the tiny energy-producing factories inside the cells). This impaired ability to burn fatty acids, either induced or inherent, helps explain why some individuals who are not overweight but who have a family history of type 2 diabetes have also been found to have fat deposits in their muscle cells.

As I mentioned previously, these fat deposits in the muscles interfere with the action of insulin in several different ways. First, they interfere directly with various insulin-signaling and glucose transport mechanisms in the muscles, reducing their ability to respond to insulin properly in metabolizing fuels such as amino acids and glucose. Second, the fat deposits also trigger the production of highly reactive oxygen molecules such as free radicals, which can also interfere with insulin signaling—an aspect of insulin resistance I discuss in detail in Strategy Chapter 8. And finally, these fat deposits can trigger inflammation inside the muscles, which also interferes with insulin action. (This inflammatory effect is in addition to the impact of obesity-related inflammation, described next.)

YOUR FAT STORES PRODUCE PRO-INFLAMMATORY SUBSTANCES THAT INTERFERE WITH INSULIN'S ACTION AND CAN ALSO DAMAGE THE PANCREAS.

Until fairly recently, fat was thought to be a passive body tissue that existed to store excess calories for later use in times of scarcity. Today, however, we know that fat tissue is very active biologically, producing many different substances that influence a wide range of metabolic processes, including the immune system's inflammatory response. When your body fat is at a healthy level, your fat stores actually work to prevent inflammation by secreting mainly anti-inflammatory proteins. As a person gains weight and his or her fat cells start to become larger, however, the stress on these cells causes them to change biochemically. As a result, they begin secreting mostly *pro-inflammatory* proteins and also attract other substances known as macrophages, which are also potent stimulators of inflammation.

In many people with supersized fat cells, this leads to a chronic state of inflammation within their fat tissues. In addition to this inflammation in the fat stores themselves, the inflammatory signals produced by these supersized fat cells also move into the bloodstream, activating other pro-inflammatory substances there, which then circulate to distant organs, causing what's known as systemic inflammation—a widespread, low-level inflammation throughout the body. Unlike acute inflammation—in which your body tissue becomes inflamed and swollen, for example, or an organ becomes painful or clearly dysfunctional—systemic chronic inflammation has no immediately apparent symptoms. But the continual activity of low levels of pro-inflammatory chemicals coursing through your bloodstream can have a wide range of negative effects on your blood vessels and other organs. Among other things, systemic inflammation is now considered a significant contributor to cardiovascular disease and has been linked to increased risk of heart attack, stroke, and hypertension. It is also emerging as a key factor in diabetes risk because we now know that inflammation causes insulin resistance and also damages the beta cells of the pancreas.

This insulin resistance is linked to the fact that pro-inflammatory proteins associated with chronic inflammation interfere with the insulin-signaling process on the cellular level. Proteins that appear to play a role in this process include the cytokines (cell-signaling proteins) tumor necrosis factor alpha (abbreviated as TNFα), interleukin-6 (IL-6), and interleukin-1 beta (IL-1β). One effect of this interference is that your body's large fat deposits become insulin resistant. Since one of insulin's actions is to stop the breakdown of fat stores and encourage fatty acids to be stored as fat instead, this loss of insulin sensitivity means your fat stores will now metabolize fat more readily and release more fatty acids into the bloodstream—leading to still more fat deposits and insulin resistance in the muscles and other peripheral tissues, as we just saw.

In addition, the systemic inflammation caused by excess body fat can contribute directly to insulin resistance in the muscles and liver, and can also damage the beta cells of the pancreas, impairing their ability to produce insulin. As I discuss in more depth in Strategy Chapter 5, systemic inflammation from obesity and other causes is now considered to be a significant contributor to increased risk for type 2 diabetes. Think of it as a silent anti-insulin agent circulating through your body, blocking the ability of your insulin to do its job and at the same time attacking the organ that produces your body's insulin.

BEING OVERWEIGHT INCREASES THE RISK OF DEVELOPING A FATTY LIVER, WHICH IN TURN LEADS TO INCREASED GLUCOSE PRODUCTION.

High levels of body fat, especially visceral abdominal fat, are also associated with fat accumulation inside the liver, due to the same increased flux of fatty acids that leads to accumulation of fat deposits inside the muscles. This fat accumulation causes the liver to become insulin resistant, due in part to the inflammatory effects of the fat buildup. Unlike the skeletal muscles, however, which either burn glucose or store it

Inside Joslin: Discovering the "Master Switch" for Obesity-Related Inflammation

In a 2005 publication, Joslin scientists reported on a pivotal study linking insulin resistance to elevated blood levels of a pro-inflammatory protein called NF-kβ, which is produced in greater amounts in people who are overweight. When they used genetic techniques to activate this protein in the livers of lean animals, raising blood levels of NF-kβ to about three times normal levels, they were able to create a widespread state of low-grade inflammation that quickly led to increased levels of insulin and blood glucose in their subjects—a clear sign that insulin resistance had set in. Our researchers are now investigating this "master switch" for inflammation to see if drugs that suppress its activity could offer a way of treating insulin resistance. For more on this research, see Strategy Chapter 5.

to be used as fuel later, the liver stores and also *produces* glucose. One important effect of insulin on the liver is to slow down the liver's glucose production and instead encourage it to store glucose as blood glucose levels rise following a meal or snack. When the liver becomes insulin resistant, this natural suppressive effect is inhibited. As a result, the liver continues churning out glucose even when blood glucose levels are elevated, further adding to the body's glucose load.

For this reason and perhaps others that haven't yet been uncovered, researchers have found that fatty liver significantly heightens the risk of type 2 diabetes. A 2011 study published in the *Journal of Clinical Endocrinology & Metabolism*, for example, found that people with fatty liver were five times more likely to develop type 2 diabetes over a five-year period than those without fatty liver.

Conversely, insulin resistance and type 2 diabetes can also *cause* fatty liver: As mentioned previously, one of insulin's actions is to process fatty acids into complex fat. When insulin levels are elevated due to insulin resistance, this effect can lead to the development of more fatty deposits in the liver. Fatty liver due to insulin resistance and diabetes is now one of the most common liver problems in this country.

Why Belly Fat Is Especially Bad for You

L eaving aside your body's small deposits of brown fat—a unique, diabetes-fighting type of fat that I discuss in detail in Strategy Chapter 4—virtually all the fat in your body consists of so-called white fat. This fat (which is actually on the yellowish side) is divided into two categories: subcutaneous fat, which generally lies beneath the skin and can be grabbed with your fingers, and visceral fat, which lies deep inside the abdomen, surrounding and cushioning your internal organs.

Although your abdomen also contains a fair amount of subcutaneous fat, most belly fat is visceral fat. Current research strongly suggests that *excess visceral fat is the primary cause of weight-related insulin resistance and type 2 diabetes.* This is likely due in part to the fact that visceral fat secretes higher levels of the fat-related pro-inflammatory chemicals that disrupt insulin's action. In addition, visceral fat appears to release fatty acids in the bloodstream more readily than subcutaneous fat. As mentioned earlier in this chapter, the increased availability of these fatty acids appears to be a key factor in the development of obesity-related insulin resistance in the skeletal muscles and liver. This relationship has been borne out by studies showing that high levels of abdominal fat are linked to elevated levels of fatty acids inside skeletal muscle. Larger amounts of abdominal fat have also been linked to increased likelihood of having fatty liver.

Although additional research is needed to pin down these mechanisms, studies have clearly established an association between abdominal fat and insulin resistance. In fact, studies have found that increased amounts of abdominal fat are associated with increased levels of insulin resistance *regardless* of whether someone is actually obese or not. This may help explain why some people, including those whose parents were both diagnosed with type 2 diabetes as well as many individuals of Asian descent, tend to develop diabetes at relatively low BMI levels: It could be that they are genetically predisposed to gain fat in their abdominal cavity, leaving them at increased risk of insulin resistance even when they aren't significantly overweight.

This is why people who are "apple" shaped (with large fat deposits in their abdomen) are at greater risk for developing type 2 diabetes than people who are "pear" shaped, meaning most of their fat is of the subcutaneous variety in their hips, buttocks, and thighs. And diabetes isn't the only medical condition associated with abdominal fat: Waist circumference and waist-to-hip ratio measurements are also used to assess risk for both cardiovascular disease and metabolic syndrome—a constellation of symptoms that can include excess abdominal fat, high blood pressure, elevated blood glucose, elevated blood triglycerides, and abnormally low levels of HDL ("good") cholesterol. In women, excessive visceral fat is also associated with increased risk of breast cancer and the need for gallbladder surgery.

America's Obesity Epidemic

According to the NHANES (National Health and Nutrition Examination Survey) data collected from their 2009–2010 cohort, 35.7% of Americans ages twenty or older—78 million adults in all—are

At-a-Glance Weight-Loss Chart

YOUR CURRENT WEIGHT IS . . .	5% TO 7% LOSS IS . . .	YOUR NEW WEIGHT . . .
120 lbs.	6 to 8 lbs.	112 to 114 lbs.
140 lbs.	7 to 10 lbs.	130 to 133 lbs.
160 lbs.	8 to 11 lbs.	149 to 152 lbs.
180 lbs.	9 to 13 lbs.	167 to 171 lbs.
200 lbs.	10 to 14 lbs.	186 to 190 lbs.
220 lbs.	11 to 15 lbs.	205 to 209 lbs.
240 lbs.	12 to 17 lbs.	223 to 228 lbs.
260 lbs.	13 to 18 lbs.	242 to 247 lbs.
280 lbs.	14 to 20 lbs.	260 to 266 lbs.
300 lbs.	15 to 21 lbs.	279 to 285 lbs.
320 lbs.	16 to 22 lbs.	298 to 304 lbs.
340 lbs.	17 to 24 lbs.	316 to 323 lbs.

now obese, defined as having a BMI of 30 or above. About one fifth of this group fall into the category of extreme obesity, defined as having a BMI of 40 or above. Another 33.1% of adult Americans are in the less dangerous overweight category, with BMIs between 25 and 30.

These statistics add up to the fact that an astonishing 68.8% of Americans—more than two thirds of our nation's adult population—are either obese or overweight. Adult obesity rates are even higher among the subgroups of Hispanic Americans (39.1%) and African Americans (49.8%). The American epidemic of excess body fat extends to our youngsters as well. Among U.S. children and adolescents ages two to nineteen, 16.9% are obese—a total of 12 million children.

The last two decades of the twentieth century was the period when obesity rates really skyrocketed in the United States. Over this time, the nation's adult obesity rate doubled from 15% in 1980 to 30.5% in the 1999–2000 NHANES survey. Since 2000, U.S. obesity rates have risen more slowly, particularly over the past several years. Between 2000 and 2010, adult obesity increased from 30.5% to 35.7%, largely due to the rise in the obesity rate of American men over that period, from 27.5% to 35.5%. During that same ten-year period, the increase in the obesity rate for U.S. women was relatively small, from 33.4% to 35.8%. As a result, the obesity gap between men and women that existed in 2000 has now vanished.

Although the rates for adult obesity in the United States may be increasing more slowly, they are still continuing to rise. In 2012, the CDC released a study projecting that if current trends hold, 42% of adult Americans will be obese by 2030.

How Did Our Country Get So Fat? Portion Sizes, Soft Drinks, and Antibiotics May Share the Blame

The causes of obesity include a wide range of genetic, biological, behavioral, cultural, and socioeconomic factors. That said, the immediate reason that anyone becomes overfat is due to a basic energy imbalance: Whenever someone takes in more calories per day than he or she is expending through physical and metabolic activity, these extra calories are stored as body fat.

Although there is clearly a genetic component to obesity—researchers recently identified six genetic variants that appear to influence BMI—it accounts for a very small percentage of the overall problem. Here are some of the other likely culprits.

INCREASED PORTION SIZES AND MORE FAST FOOD

According to the National Institutes of Health, the caloric content of portions served by American restaurants has more than doubled over the past twenty years. Over this same time period, the percentage of daily calories that Americans get from calorie-dense fast food has risen from 2% to 10%.

CONSUMPTION OF SUGAR-SWEETENED BEVERAGES

Americans' overall energy intake from sweetened beverages increased by 135% from 1977 until 2001, resulting in an average daily increase of 278 calories per person. The main sweeteners, sucrose (table sugar) and high-fructose corn syrup, are combinations of glucose and fructose—both high in calories with no nutritional value. Fructose is especially problematic because the liver processes it into fat. Another problem is that our satiety mechanisms don't register the calories delivered through these liquids—making it easy to overconsume calories when these beverages are a regular part of meals. One study found that U.S. adolescents get 11% of their daily calories from sugar-rich soft drinks.

PHYSICAL INACTIVITY

Although the role of physical activity, or the lack thereof, in America's obesity epidemic seems like a no-brainer, the evidence for this being a driving factor is actually mixed. A number of studies have found that people who report engaging in the least physical activity are the most likely to experience significant weight gain over time. To some extent, decreased physical activity may also have contributed to increases in childhood obesity. For example, studies have linked weight gain in youngsters to time spent on sedentary activities such as watching TV and playing video games. It is not, however, clear from large-scale studies whether overall physical inactivity among children is actually linked to weight gain.

CHANGES IN OUR INTESTINAL BACTERIA DUE TO OVERUSE OF ANTIBIOTICS

Recent research on the microbiome—the term used to describe the billions of different bacteria that live inside our bodies, especially in our intestinal tracts—suggests that Americans' widespread exposure to antibiotics, particularly from the administration of these drugs to the livestock we eat to promote growth, may be contributing to the obesity epidemic as well: Exposure of adults to low-level antibiotics over a period of time has been linked to an increase in BMI, presumably because it causes a shift in intestinal bacteria toward a mix that is more efficient at extracting calories from the food we eat. Similar to microbiome studies in adults, researchers have also linked antibiotic use in infancy to increased risk of childhood obesity.

Losing Weight: A Proven Way to Prevent Diabetes

Just as we now have convincing research showing that excess body fat can contribute to insulin resistance and type 2 diabetes risk, there is also strong evidence that losing even a relatively modest amount of fat can significantly improve your blood glucose metabolism—presumably by shrinking your fat cells to the point where their production of fatty acids and inflammatory cytokines is substantially reduced. Two landmark studies conducted over the past decade, the Diabetes Prevention Program and the Look AHEAD Study, have both shown that losing 5% to 7% of one's body weight is enough to significantly improve the body's ability to metabolize blood glucose and can also delay or prevent the onset of type 2 diabetes.

THE DIABETES PREVENTION PROGRAM

The Diabetes Prevention Program (DPP) was a federally funded, multicenter study that began in the late 1990s. Its 3,234 subjects were all overweight and had prediabetes at the time they were enrolled, putting them at high risk for developing diabetes. The participants were divided into three groups. One group received intensive lifestyle counseling aimed at helping them lose 7% of their body weight by reducing their daily intake of dietary fat and total calories and walking the equivalent of thirty minutes a day, five days per week. Another group was given standard information on diet and exercise plus a daily dose of the diabetes medication metformin. The third group got standard information on diet and exercise and a placebo pill in place of metformin.

The study, which published its results in 2002 in the *New England Journal of Medicine*, found that the group receiving intensive lifestyle counseling lost an average of fifteen pounds over a year's time and that they also reduced their risk of developing type 2 diabetes over the next three years by 58% compared to the study's placebo group. Participants who were sixty or older at the start of the study benefited even more from the weight-loss and exercise program, reducing their diabetes risk by 71% compared to their age-matched peers. Since that original publication, a follow-up study has found that these benefits were still apparent ten years after the subjects' initial time of enrollment: The lifestyle group had a 34% lower incidence of diabetes over that time period compared to the placebo group, whereas participants who were sixty or older at the start of the study had a 49% lower rate of diabetes than those receiving the placebo treatment.

THE LOOK AHEAD STUDY

The Look AHEAD Study was launched in 2001 and was originally intended to last thirteen years (AHEAD is a semi-acronym for "Action for HEAlth in Diabetes). It followed 5,145 people who had already been diagnosed with type 2 diabetes. The subjects, who had an average age of sixty and an average BMI of 36, were divided into two groups. One group received intensive lifestyle counseling on diet and exercise in the form of forty-two individual and group sessions over the first year of the study and were encouraged to reduce their starting weight by at least 10% (a goal chosen in hopes of achieving a group-wide average weight reduction of at least 7%). The lifestyle intervention also included an exercise target consisting of 175 minutes of moderately intense activity per week (25 minutes a day), which was somewhat more ambitious than the DPP's exercise plan. The second group, meanwhile, received just three basic Diabetes Support and Education (DSE) sessions.

Inside Joslin: Our Own Weight-Loss Success Story

Joslin's weight-loss program has produced some of the field's best results in terms of consistent weight loss and improved glucose control among large groups of people previously diagnosed with diabetes or prediabetes. Our intensive twelve-week program employs a combination of techniques, including a reduced-calorie eating plan and individualized exercise plans. Participants also receive cognitive behavioral support through sessions with a clinical psychologist, addressing issues such as self-monitoring of eating and exercise, behavioral goal setting, overcoming negative thinking patterns, assertive communication skills, stress management, and relapse prevention.

In 2008, Joslin published a study of five different groups that went through our twelve-week weight-loss course. This study found that:

- Participants lost an average of 10% of their initial weight (an average of 23.5 pounds) and 3.5 inches from their waistlines.

- Average hemoglobin A1C measurements of participants decreased almost 10%, from 7.26 to 6.37.

- Participants' total cholesterol decreased an average of 12%, including an 11% drop in LDL cholesterol, while triglyceride levels decreased by 22% on average.

- C-reactive protein (CRP) levels (a marker for systemic inflammation) decreased from 6.0 to 4.2 on average, a drop of 30%.

Participants in the Joslin weight-loss program were also able to significantly reduce the amounts of diabetes drugs they were taking, resulting in an average savings of $561 per year on diabetes medications. A number of participants who had been on insulin therapy were able to stop taking insulin completely, while the rest were able to cut their daily doses of both long-acting and short-acting insulin by more than 50%.

Even more important, a large majority of participants were able to avoid regaining the weight they had lost, to a great extent—a goal that very few weight-loss programs have been able to achieve. One year after completing the Joslin program, the group as a whole reported they had regained an average of just 5.3 pounds each from their lowest weight—meaning they had continued to maintain an average weight loss of 18.2 pounds, or 7.6% of their initial body weight. In addition, more than half the study group continued to lose additional weight in the year following their participation in the Joslin program.

In 2013, four-year follow-up data from the Joslin weight-loss study were presented at the annual meeting of the American Association of Diabetes Educators. Of the 119 patients that the study had continued to track, 57 had managed to maintain their entire weight loss after four years, recording an average reduction of twenty-four pounds since entering the Joslin weight-loss program.

Participants in the lifestyle group also got in-depth counseling on portion control and were encouraged to replace two meals and one snack each day with meal-replacement shakes and bars over the first six months of the study. During the second six months, they were encouraged to continue substituting a meal-replacement shake for one meal per day. Those who hadn't reached their interim weight-loss goals at that point were also provided with a "toolbox" designed to help them identify and address problem behaviors that were interfering with their weight-loss program.

By the end of the study's first year, the difference between the effectiveness of the two approaches was abundantly clear. The lifestyle intervention group had reduced their starting weight by 8.7% on average, whereas the DSE group had lost just .7% of their initial weight. The intervention group also recorded a 21% increase in aerobic fitness and their average hemoglobin A1C levels dropped from 7.3 to 6.6.

Following that first year, the intervention group continued to receive individualized support and regular invitations to participate in motivational campaigns over the next three years. (After that three-year follow-up period was over, they continued to have access to monthly onsite visits as well as yearly refresher courses to help them maintain weight loss.) In the study's four-year follow-up, published in 2010, the lifestyle intervention group was able to maintain an average weight reduction of 6% below their starting weight. They had also maintained a 12% improvement in fitness, an average drop of .36 in their hemoglobin A1C levels, and significant reductions in their blood pressure and trigylceride levels.

Interestingly, the study was ended two years early after it was found that this reduction in weight and other risk factors did not translate into lower heart attack or stroke rates among the intervention group. Their changes in lifestyle did, however, provide clear diabetes-related health benefits, including a reduced need for diabetes medications.

Both the DPP and the Look AHEAD Study also offered valuable insights into what weight-reduction techniques work best in a multidisciplinary setting. Joslin clinicians drew on the approaches used in these studies when we designed Joslin's highly regarded weight-loss

program—the world's first clinical practice program designed
specifically to help patients with
diabetes lose weight through a
novel multidisciplinary approach.
By employing a more focused
approach to counseling and group
support than the DPP and Look
AHEAD Study, we've been able to
achieve even more robust results
in terms of sustained weight loss.
(See box on page 89: Inside Joslin:
Our Own Weight-Loss Success
Story.)

Ten Essential Tips for Losing Weight

One of the most important
things we've learned is that
for a weight-loss program to work,
it must be multidimensional,
addressing what you eat, how and

> ### The Twenty to Twenty-Five Plan: An Alternative Approach to Calorie Restriction
>
> If you want to take a more extended approach to weight loss without restricting calories as severely, try following a regimen of twenty to twenty-five daily calories per kilogram (2.2 pounds) of body weight, which for a moderately active person typically results in a slight negative energy imbalance (meaning you will be burning a few more calories each day than you're taking in). For a 200-pound person, this translates to a range of 1,815 to 2,270 calories per day. To find the lower limit of your own daily calorie range using this approach, multiply your weight in pounds by 9.1; to find the upper limit, multiply your weight by 11.35.

where you consume your food, your level of physical activity, your support system, and any psychological barriers that may be impeding your
weight loss.

1. AIM TO LOSE A TARGETED AMOUNT OF WEIGHT OVER A PERIOD OF THREE TO SIX MONTHS BY FOLLOWING A CALORIE-RESTRICTED EATING PLAN.

Because sticking to a calorie-restricted eating plan—which is the centerpiece of any successful weight-loss program—is inherently difficult, the
most successful weight-loss regimens ask participants to significantly
reduce their calorie intake for a limited amount of time, after which
time they can relax their calorie restriction. During this initial period,

they are encouraged to aim for a steady, consistent rate of weight loss that will bring them to a certain target weight by the end of the calorie restriction period. Once the target weight is reached, calorie restriction can be eased, as the emphasis switches to maintenance. At the same time, consuming fewer daily calories will hopefully have become more habitual at this point.

The DPP employed a twenty-four-week weight-loss curriculum, during which participants were encouraged to reduce their starting weight by at least 7%. The Look AHEAD Study followed a similar approach, aiming for a six-month weight-reduction period, during which participants would try to lose 7% or more of their body weight. The researchers noted that they chose this amount of time rather than a longer, one-year

Counting Calories? There's an App for That

There are several popular smartphone apps for tracking calorie and nutrient intake, and we're listing the three we think are best. They're all free downloads and follow the same basic approach: They ask you to enter a personal profile, including your weight-loss goal and daily calorie limits, then let you quickly search out the caloric and nutritional content of any food item you're planning to consume, record how many calories you consume per meal and per day, check how many of your daily calories you've used up at any point in time, and track your progress toward your goals.

Lose It!

This easy-to-use iPhone and Android app contains a comprehensive database of foods, with detailed information on their calories and nutritional content. It provides daily menu templates that let you calculate and record intake for each meal and also lets you calculate and log calories expended in physical activity.

MyFitnessPal Calorie Counter and Fitness Tracker

This app is available for the iPhone, Android, BlackBerry, and Windows Phone. In addition to a database of more than seven hundred thousand foods, it offers a barcode scanner that lets you quickly analyze the nutritional information in packaged foods and includes a function to log and record exercise calories burned.

MyNetDiary Calorie Counter

This app, available for iPhone and Android phones, provides calorie and nutrition information on more than four hundred thousand foods, allowing you to log daily meals and workouts.

period because "mean weight loss generally plateaus at six months with all [nonsurgical] interventions."

The Joslin weight-loss program has found that comparable reductions in weight can be obtained over a more concentrated twelve-week period, during which participants aim for a weight loss of 7% or more. This twelve-week period includes intermediate goals of a 3% reduction in weight by the end of week four and a 5% reduction by the end of week eight. In Part Two of *The Diabetes Reset*, I'll provide a schedule that you can use to implement your own weight-loss plan.

2. REDUCE YOUR DAILY CALORIE INTAKE BY ABOUT 500 CALORIES DURING YOUR TARGETED WEIGHT-LOSS PERIOD.

At the start of Joslin's twelve-week weight-loss program, all participants are evaluated by a registered dietitian who reviews their dietary history and also has them do a twenty-four-hour recall of a typical day's intake of food. Based on the calories consumed in this typical daily eating pattern, participants are then given a meal plan that reduces their daily energy intake by 500 calories, rounded to the nearest 1,200, 1,500, or

The Importance of Portion Control

One of the simplest ways to cut your daily caloric intake is to reduce the portion size of the foods you eat and also be prepared to leave some of that food uneaten on your plate. A steady increase in the size of the food portions consumed by Americans appears to be a prime contributor to our nation's obesity epidemic: In a nationwide study that looked at changes in food consumption patterns from 1977 to 1998, researchers found that portion sizes increased significantly over that time for a range of high-calorie foods, including salty snacks (an average per-portion increase of 93 calories more), soft drinks (49 calories), hamburgers (97 calories), French fries (68 calories), and Mexican dishes (133 calories).

Researchers have also shown that when people are given larger portions of food, they invariably eat more of that food. In one experiment using four different serving sizes of macaroni and cheese, for example, those given the largest-size servings consumed an average of 30% more calories per serving than those given portions half that size.

1,800 calorie level. In practice, the vast majority of the men in the Joslin program end up starting with a diet plan based on consuming 1,800 calories per day, and most women start on a 1,500-calorie diet plan.

3. MONITOR AND RECORD YOUR DAILY AND WEEKLY CALORIC INTAKE.

As I noted earlier, the key to losing weight is to change your energy balance and begin burning more energy than you take in each day. In order to do this, it is essential that you control the amount of calories you take in—and this means being aware of how many calories you are consuming every time you eat. There are a number of free smartphone apps that help you to determine the amount of calories in different serving sizes of a wide variety of foods, including restaurant offerings, and track the number of calories you consume in each meal. (See box on page 92: Counting Calories? There's an App for That.) I strongly recommend that you download one of these and begin using it on a regular basis. Studies have shown that the more often people record their food intake, the greater the weight reduction they are able to achieve and maintain.

4. MAKE SURE THAT YOUR CALORIE-RESTRICTED DIET INCLUDES A HEALTHY BALANCE OF COMPLEX CARBOHYDRATES, FAT (PRIMARILY UNSATURATED FAT), PROTEIN, AND FIBER.

In addition to having a firm idea of the number of calories you're taking in, you will need to expend your allotted daily calories on a mix of foods that will optimize your body's metabolic activity while also providing a sense of being satiated. I recommend following the low-fat, high-fiber Rural Asian Diet (RAD) eating plan outlined in the preceding chapter. My own research has identified this approach as a highly effective diet for reversing and preventing type 2 diabetes. Our clinical trial of this diet found that it encourages weight loss even without any calorie restriction, but you can also use this eating plan as the foundation of your own personalized weight-loss program by incorporating it into a targeted period in which you limit your caloric intake. You can also combine the Rural Asian Diet with meal replacement products designed to encourage weight loss, as described in Weight-Loss Tip 6 that follows.

I should note that the nutrient mix of the RAD eating plan—70% carbohydrates, 15% protein, and 15% fat—differs considerably from nutrient ratios of low-carb weight-loss programs, which typically utilize a mix of around 40% carbohydrates, 30% protein, and 30% fat. I firmly believe that although these kinds of low-carb, high-protein, and high-fat diets can be effective at promoting weight loss over a period of three to six months, you are best off embarking now on an eating plan like the Rural Asian Diet that can be sustained for a lifetime and that will help optimize your glucose metabolism and cardiovascular health from Day One.

5. WEIGH YOURSELF OFTEN—DAILY, IF POSSIBLE, AND AT LEAST WEEKLY—TO TRACK YOUR PROGRESS DURING YOUR WEIGHT-REDUCTION PHASE AND TO AVOID REGAINING WEIGHT LATER.

Numerous studies have found that the more often people engaged in weight-reduction programs weigh themselves, the more weight they lose. For example, a 2007 study analyzing three thousand members of the National Weight Control Registry, all of whom had lost thirty or more pounds and maintained this weight loss for at least one year, found that

Portion Sizes at a Glance

A SERVING IN THIS AMOUNT . . .	IS THE SIZE OF . . .
1 cup of fruit, salad greens	A baseball
½ cup of cooked grains, pasta, or vegetables	Half a baseball
3.5 ounces of meat or poultry	A deck of playing cards
3.5 ounces of fish	A large-screen smartphone
1.5 ounces of cheese	2 slices or 4 dice cubes
2 tablespoons of dip or spread	1 Ping-Pong ball

those who weighed themselves at least once a day had lower BMIs and higher scores on behavior scales associated with successful weight loss than those who weighed themselves less often.

6. ENGAGE IN A STRUCTURED PROGRAM OF PHYSICAL ACTIVITY THAT INVOLVES AT LEAST 150 MINUTES OF MODERATE EXERCISE PER WEEK.

Although exercise alone usually won't tilt your energy balance enough to produce significant weight loss, research shows that a regular program of daily exercise dramatically improves your chances of losing weight and keeping the pounds off through calorie restriction. In Strategy Chapter 3, I will outline a research-based exercise program that can easily be incorporated into your weight-loss plan and that will also boost your insulin sensitivity on its own, independent of any weight you lose.

As noted previously, participants in the Diabetes Prevention Program were encouraged to get at least 150 minutes of moderate exercise each week, whereas Look AHEAD participants were given a goal of 175 minutes of weekly exercise. The Look AHEAD Study found that the quartile of participants who reported the highest level of physical activity—averaging nearly five hours of exercise each week—also had the greatest reduction in weight, recording an average weight loss of 11.7%.

There have also been recent discussions in the diabetes research community about whether short periods of intensive exercise may be just as good as longer, more moderate exercise at improving insulin resistance. It is not clear how long the beneficial effects of these short bursts will last, however, and the physiological effects of short-duration, high-intensity exercise also place greater stress on the heart than the exercise program outlined in this book. For these reasons, my recommendation is still to do twenty-five minutes of moderate exercise per day—the amount of time it takes to watch a situation comedy or the evening news on TV.

To give your workouts an extra energy-burning boost, recent findings suggest that exercising in temperatures of 68°F or cooler will also activate your brown fat stores, enabling you to expend even more calories than you would exercising at temperatures of 68°F or more. (For more on the remarkable calorie-burning qualities of brown fat, see Strategy Chapter 4.)

As mentioned previously, in addition to its impact on weight loss, a program of daily exercise will also act directly to improve insulin sensitivity in the skeletal muscles. I discuss these important benefits in detail in Strategy Chapter 3 and explain why regular physical activity is an essential tool for preventing or reversing insulin resistance and type 2 diabetes.

7. DEVELOP A PERSONALIZED WEIGHT-LOSS STRATEGY THAT INCLUDES IDENTIFYING AND MODIFYING YOUR OWN BEHAVIORAL BARRIERS TO WEIGHT LOSS.

Weight-loss research has shown that people who are successful at losing a desired amount of weight tend to develop individualized strategies designed to help them overcome their own personal barriers to weight

What a Successful Weight-Loss Mind-Set Looks Like

Researchers have found that people who manage to lose a significant amount of weight and keep it off tend to have a number of traits in common. These include:

- Being honest with themselves at all times

- Placing a healthy value on their own needs and desires

- Recognizing that changing long-held behaviors requires hard work and persistence

- Starting to work on their goals now instead of waiting for a "better" or "ideal" time

- Tailoring various weight-loss approaches to their own lifestyle

- Taking personal responsibility for the changes they need to make rather than relying on someone else

- Viewing weight loss as part of a long-term growth and learning process and not an end in itself

- Trusting themselves and realizing that it's okay to slip up and learn from their mistakes

- Following a flexible, incremental approach in which they progress one step at a time, building on small successes, rather than trying to be "perfect"

- Taking ownership of their own successes and slip-ups rather than seeking approval from others

The Importance of Assertive Communication

Because a program of healthy eating and exercise may entail making specific requests for certain foods and modes of preparation and also involves setting aside time for physical activity, successful weight loss requires learning to stand up for your own needs by developing assertive communication skills. It's a fact of life that other people are not always going to be as cooperative as you'd like them to be in helping you stick to your eating or exercise plan. They may simply be inattentive or distracted, or they may not care as much as you do, or they may be uncomfortable with or resistant to the idea of helping you achieve a healthier eating pattern and lifestyle.

Learning to communicate assertively around eating and lifestyle situations includes identifying your own barriers to assertive communication—you may be reluctant to "make a fuss," for example, or you may be concerned that you'll be viewed as too demanding. You want to be *assertive* about your goals by stating them clearly, pleasantly, and calmly. You want to avoid being *aggressive* about your goals—that is, accusatory or making the other person feel defensive or in the wrong. And you also should avoid being *passive*, in which you simply give in rather than ask for assistance.

Here are some guidelines for communicating your needs in a positive, assertive way:

• Stick to the facts of the situation rather than make assumptions about the other person's motivations.

• Rather than making the other person "wrong," keep the focus on your own feelings by using "I" statements rather than "you" statements.

• Focus on the specific behavior you'd like to see happen.

• When asking for what you want, maintain a friendly, calm, but firm tone of voice.

• Don't be afraid to keep repeating your needs or desires until they're acknowledged.

Examples

At a restaurant: "I'm sorry, but I'd asked for brown rice in place of the French fries. Could you please bring the correct order?"

At work: "Can we try serving fruit instead of pastries at our breakfast meetings?"

With friends: "I'd love to set up a time each week when we can meet to go walking together."

With family: "Your homemade fudge looks delicious and I wish I could have some, but I'm trying to lose weight, so I'll have to pass."

loss. Cognitive-behavioral counseling, in which patients are encouraged to identify and modify patterns of thinking linked to nonconstructive behaviors, have been found to be especially effective at encouraging weight loss.

During the twelve-week weight-reduction phase of Joslin's weight-loss program, participants attend weekly group behavioral support sessions led by a clinical psychologist. During these sessions, participants learn a number of cognitive-behavioral techniques adapted from the Diabetes Prevention Program. These include:

- Developing a new style of preparing and eating food that employs healthier food choices and significantly smaller amounts of food
- Deemphasizing the importance of food in your life
- Setting small, attainable goals
- Persisting in new eating patterns until you develop a sense of personal ownership in them and they become your "new normal"
- Developing strategies other than eating for coping with stressful situations

Finally, it's important to stick to your plan and not be discouraged by the many different tips and strategies for losing weight that you'll encounter in the media. People can and do lose weight through the approaches outlined in this chapter—and you can, too.

8. CONSIDER USING MEAL REPLACEMENT PRODUCTS DURING YOUR ACUTE WEIGHT-LOSS PHASE.

Although meal replacement shakes and bars aren't for everyone, they have been found to significantly increase weight loss in a number of studies involving structured weight-loss programs. Meal replacement products customized for optimal glucose control are considered to be an especially valuable component in weight-loss programs for people with diabetes or impaired glucose tolerance. They contain a fixed number of calories and a carefully calibrated blend of carbohydrates, fat, and protein designed to maximize feelings of satiety while minimizing the rise in blood glucose after eating, making it easier for those using them to keep total caloric intake within daily targets. I should note that their mix of nutrients diverges significantly from the mix found in the RAD eating plan outlined in Strategy Chapter 1—but if these products, used over a short period of time, are able to help you lose weight where other weight-loss strategies fail, then you should consider using them.

In Joslin's weight-loss program, participants are instructed to use a nutritionally complete meal replacement shake for both breakfast and lunch during at least the first six weeks of the program. The meal replacement we use is BOOST® Glucose Control™ from Nestlé Medical Nutrition, Inc., which can be purchased for home use as well. The Look AHEAD Study also instructed participants to use meal replacement shakes for breakfast and lunch and to eat a meal replacement bar as a daily snack over a seventeen-week period. They offered their participants a choice of several meal replacement products tailored to people with impaired glucose control, including Slimfast (Unilever), Glucerna (Abbott Laboratories), and HMR (Health Management Resources Corporation).

Should You Enroll in a Formal Weight-Loss Program?

Research shows that although joining a formal weight-loss program can be helpful, it's not absolutely necessary. Among the members of the National Weight Control Registry— members of a large-scale study, all of whom have lost 30% or more of their body weight and kept that weight off for at least a year—a little more than half (55%) achieved their weight loss by participating in a formal program, while 45% shed their excess pounds on their own. If you are thinking of enrolling in a weight-loss program, I would urge you to consider a program designed specifically for people with glucose control issues, such as Joslin's weight-loss program (which is offered at our Boston clinic) or one of the hundreds of nationally accredited Diabetes Prevention Programs (DPPs) available across the nation. A state-by-state registry of DPP can be found on the website of the Centers for Disease Control and Prevention at: cdc.gov/diabetes/prevention/recognition/registry.htm.

Bariatric Surgery: A Shortcut That Appears to Work

Although *The Diabetes Reset* is focused on ways you can improve your insulin sensitivity without medication or surgery, any chapter on diabetes-related weight loss would be remiss not to point out that for people who are unable to lose weight through calorie restriction and exercise alone, bariatric surgery—including gastric bypass, gastric band, and sleeve gastrectomy procedures—has proven to be an effective alternative in terms of both losing weight and improving blood glucose control.

In a groundbreaking clinical trial at the Cleveland Clinic, the results of which were published in 2012 in the *New England Journal of Medicine*, 150 obese patients with uncontrolled type 2 diabetes were randomly assigned to receive either intensive medical therapy or a gastric bypass or sleeve gastrectomy stomach reduction operation. When they enrolled in the study, the subjects were taking an average of three diabetes medications each. Twelve months after the start of treatment, 43% of the bypass group and 37% of the sleeve surgery group had hemoglobin A1C levels below 6.0, which is considered a normal blood glucose level, compared to just 12% of those undergoing medical therapy. Every member of the bypass group who reached this level did so without medication, whereas 72% of the sleeve therapy group reached the

normal level without drugs. Overall, the bypass group lost an average of sixty-five pounds each, whereas the sleeve group lost an average of fifty-five pounds.

At this time, the International Diabetes Federation recommends bariatric surgery for people with type 2 diabetes who have a BMI greater than 35 or a BMI between 30 and 35 with diabetes that cannot be controlled by medication and lifestyle changes. Although it's my belief—backed up, as this book shows, by clinical research—that most people with prediabetes or type 2 diabetes can improve their condition significantly through lifestyle changes and, where needed, medication, it will be interesting to follow the continuing refinement of these bariatric procedures and the benefits they offer in terms of long-term glucose control for people who don't respond to other treatment approaches.

One thing to be aware of is that there are clear side effects associated with bariatric surgery, and these operations need to be carefully planned to avoid or minimize post-surgical complications. Although the more extensive bariatric procedures produce better outcomes in terms of weight loss, they also have more side effects, including gastrointestinal distress, absorption problems, and nutritional deficiencies.

9. ONCE YOU'VE ACHIEVED YOUR DESIRED WEIGHT LOSS, TRANSITION TO A WEIGHT-MAINTENANCE PROGRAM.

Studies show that a program of regular physical activity is one of the key components for keeping excess pounds off once you've lost them. And although you can raise your calorie intake by 500 calories per day once you've reached your weight-loss goal, it's also important to continue following a diet low in saturated fats and high in complex carbohydrates and fiber. For the best results, I recommend adopting the RAD eating plan outlined in Strategy Chapter 1 as your maintenance diet.

10. DEVELOP A STRONG SUPPORT SYSTEM.

Researchers have found that strong social support, particularly from family members, is important for achieving and especially maintaining weight loss. One key step in strengthening your family support system is to identify specific things family members do to help you achieve your weight-loss and activity goals (such as bringing fresh fruit and vegetables into the home, giving positive feedback after exercise sessions, and being supportive of low-calorie restaurant options) and ways they may be hindering your efforts (bringing high-calorie foods into the home, refusing to join in daily walks, or insisting on eating at fast-food restaurants). Once you are aware of these behaviors, you can begin encouraging family members to engage in helpful behaviors and avoid unhelpful ones.

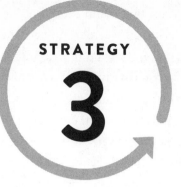

STRATEGY

3

INCREASE YOUR MUSCLES' GLUCOSE-ABSORBING ABILITY THROUGH AEROBIC EXERCISE AND STRENGTH TRAINING

The skeletal muscles—the muscles in your limbs and torso that move you through space—are responsible for burning most of the insulin-mediated glucose that your body consumes. But your muscles can lose insulin sensitivity due to physical inactivity, the accumulation of fat in the muscle tissue, and inflammation. This insulin resistance in the muscles is now considered a major cause of prediabetes and type 2 diabetes.

The good news: Skeletal muscle insulin resistance can be largely reversed through a combination of daily aerobic exercise and two or three strength training sessions per week. When done together, these activities will boost muscle insulin sensitivity dramatically by increasing your muscles' ability to oxidize fats, glucose, and other fuels. Exercise also helps your muscles metabolize glucose in another way, by activating an important noninsulin mechanism that muscle tissues use to burn glucose as fuel.

"People often talk about studying 'exercise' as if it's a special activity. But really, physical activity is the normal human state. It's what our human bodies are supposed to be doing," says Dr. Laurie Goodyear, one of the senior investigators at Joslin. "In terms of human evolution, this idea of sitting at our desks for eight hours a day is a very recent development. For most of our history, we were constantly moving."

Dr. Goodyear is the head of Joslin's Integrative Physiology and Metabolism division, known around the world for its groundbreaking discoveries about the links between exercise and diabetes. In her laboratory, the effects of physical activity are studied from every angle: The facility contains a normal-sized treadmill where human beings can walk or run while their physiological responses are measured and also has miniature treadmills and cages linked to exercise wheels, where laboratory mice can run to their heart's content. Nearby, shelves of petri dishes with cultured muscle cells are being analyzed to tease out the chemical reactions that all this exercise produces.

Thanks to the work in Dr. Goodyear's lab and others like it around the world, we are beginning to understand exactly how physical activity changes the biology of our muscles and why increasing your amount of daily physical activity is one of the keys to preventing or reversing type 2 diabetes. Their findings are helping to fill in the details of a biological fact we've known about for a while: Insulin resistance—which, as we've seen, is the main cause of both prediabetes and type 2 diabetes—*occurs largely in the muscles*. The reason is simple: Lab tests have shown that about 80% of the glucose circulating in the blood after a meal—when glucose levels spike and must be quickly metabolized—is taken up by the skeletal muscles. (In a fasting state, such as when you wake in the morning, the muscles rely much more on fat than on glucose for fuel, which is why your brain is the main utilizer of glucose at these times.) Some of the glucose taken up by the muscles is burned immediately as fuel, but most of it is stored as glycogen inside the muscles, to be broken back down into glucose and used as energy later. In people with type 2 diabetes, however, the ability of the muscles to take up glucose after a meal is reduced by *as much as one half.*

If you can change the physiology of your muscles and reverse this insulin resistance (something that can be accomplished to a large degree by losing weight and exercising), you'll be taking a major step toward restoring their glucose-absorbing ability and preventing or even reversing type 2 diabetes.

Muscles and Microscopic Fat Deposits

Although the full story of insulin resistance is complex and involves a number of contributing factors, scientists believe that one primary cause involves tiny deposits of fat that accumulate inside the muscle cells, mainly as the result of weight gain and physical inactivity. Because the fuel your muscles run on includes fatty acids, there is always some fat inside your muscle cells. In people with prediabetes and type 2 diabetes, however, the prevalence of these fat deposits (known scientifically as "intramyocellular lipids") tends to be significantly greater. Sophisticated experiments have found that these excess fat deposits interfere with insulin's ability to transport glucose into the muscle cells—leaving that glucose to circulate through your bloodstream instead.

This condition, known as insulin resistance—because the muscles have become "resistant" to the effects of insulin—requires the body to pump out more insulin in order to transport enough glucose into the muscles to keep blood glucose levels under control. As I explained in this book's introduction, people can have insulin resistance and still maintain normal blood glucose levels for years, so long as they can continue to produce enough insulin to overcome their insulin resistance and metabolize the glucose in their bloodstream. In many individuals, however, their bodies eventually become unable to produce sufficient insulin. This is especially likely to happen with people who are at heightened risk of type 2 diabetes due to obesity, a family history of diabetes, or a personal history of gestational diabetes. Over time, the beta cells of the pancreas can no longer keep pace—either because their function becomes impaired, or because the insulin resistance has become too great to overcome, or both. This leads to the chronically elevated blood glucose levels associated with prediabetes and type 2 diabetes.

By the time this happens, however, many people have already been developing insulin resistance in their muscles for ten to twenty years or more. And because insulin resistance can start causing cardiovascular disease well before the onset of prediabetes or diabetes, this means that your blood vessels are being damaged over this time as well.

Insulin resistance in the muscles is now considered to be one of the very earliest stages of the diabetes pathway. The good news is that you can begin reversing this insulin resistance in your skeletal muscles starting *now,* by becoming more physically active through a program of regular aerobic and resistance exercise.

Debunking the Media: Why More Exercise Is Better, and the "Seven-Minute Workout" Is Both Impractical and Risky for People with Diabetes

MEDIA MYTH: TO BECOME HEALTHY AND FIT, ALL YOU NEED TO DO IS ONE INTENSE SEVEN-MINUTE WORKOUT EACH DAY.
I've used the example of a "seven-minute workout" here because a high-intensity exercise routine of that length was recently a popular news subject, but there have been plenty of five-, ten-, and fifteen-minute workouts over the years that claim to do the same thing. The central problem with such workouts involves the need to maintain your effort at a *very* high intensity for the entire seven minutes. For most people reading this book, a workout that involves this kind of very intense effort is both unwise and unworkable, especially if you have diabetes. If you have not done any regular aerobic exercise in quite some time, exercising in a way that makes your heart rate soar (the seven-minute workout, for example, calls for reaching 100% of your maximum heart rate!) can seriously endanger your health. For people who have already developed diabetes, which leaves them at heightened risk for heart arrhythmias, there is a very real prospect they could suffer a fatal heart attack when attempting a workout of this sort. The seven-minute workout that has gotten media attention is so strenuous, in fact, that if you read the actual journal article the workout is based on, the authors admit that many people—even those who are quite fit—will be unable to do it at the required

intensity and recommend that most exercisers do a slightly less intense twenty-minute workout instead.

Beyond the obvious and very real health concerns of such an approach, any exercise program that requires a very intense effort every day is not an easy program to stick with. Whether you have diabetes or not, the biggest obstacle in becoming physically active is usually not starting an exercise program, but maintaining it. Research shows that the majority of people who begin an overly intense and challenging exercise plan quit within a few months. That's why *The Diabetes Reset* focuses on building up to a practical, sustainable program of regular moderate exercise that can comfortably be done anywhere, anytime.

MEDIA MYTH: ANY AEROBIC EXERCISE BEYOND TWENTY MINUTES IS A WASTE OF TIME.

Like many media myths, this one contains a morsel of truth: After twenty minutes, the calorie-burning effects of a given aerobic workout begin to diminish slightly—although you'll continue to burn substantially more calories than you would at rest during *every* minute you engage in aerobic activity. When it comes to this book's main concern, however, which is preventing or controlling type 2 diabetes, more aerobic exercise has clearly been shown to produce better results by further enhancing your mitochondrial function and also further stimulating the noninsulin glucose metabolizing effects of exercise. As you will see from the numerous, large-scale exercise studies I cite in this chapter, the evidence is unequivocal: The more total minutes of physical activity

Key Exercise Terms

AEROBIC EXERCISE. Any activity you can do for an extended period of time, such as walking, cycling, swimming, jogging, tennis, or working out on an elliptical trainer. Any type of moderately intense aerobic exercise will make your muscles more sensitive to insulin.

RESISTANCE TRAINING, also known as *STRENGTH TRAINING.* Exercises that involve lifting or moving a fairly heavy weight or other resistance such as an exercise band. When strength training is done properly, you should be able to do only a limited number of repetitions (typically eight to fifteen) before the muscles involved get too fatigued to continue.

you can put in each week, the lower your risk of developing type 2 diabetes will become—and the healthier you will be overall.

What the Research Shows

A number of large-scale studies have shown conclusively that when people with prediabetes follow this double-barreled approach—losing a modest amount of weight while significantly increasing physical activity—it sharply reduces the likelihood that they will go on to develop type 2 diabetes.

The Diabetes Prevention Program study (also discussed in the last chapter) published its results in the *New England Journal of Medicine* in 2002. The study divided more than three thousand individuals with prediabetes into three groups. One group was encouraged to lose 7% of their body weight and adopt an exercise program involving 150 minutes a week of moderate physical activity equivalent to brisk walking. A second group was put on the diabetes drug metformin, and a third control group was given "standard of care" medical attention but no intensive lifestyle guidance or medication. After three years, the group that lost weight and exercised was 58% less likely to develop diabetes compared to the control group—a significantly bigger reduction in risk than the metformin group, which was 31% less likely to get diabetes.

Although exercise can be helpful in a weight-loss program, physical activity in and of itself also provides important benefits for glucose control. A number of large-scale studies have found, for example, that people with prediabetes who exercise frequently are less likely to develop diabetes *whether or not* they lose weight. A meta-analysis of fourteen studies of exercise interventions for people with type 2 diabetes, published in 2006, found that regular exercise reduced participants' hemoglobin A1C levels by .6, on average—approaching the impact of medications on A1C levels, despite that fact that the subjects lost no weight on average. They also showed significant increases in insulin sensitivity and reductions in their blood triglyceride levels.

In another well-known study that followed six thousand male University of Pennsylvania graduates for fourteen years, researchers found that every additional 500 calories each of their research subjects expended exercising per week—the amount a 190-pound person would burn walking just five miles at a moderate pace—reduced that person's risk of developing diabetes by 6%. Note that this is *independent of all other variables.* It means that, in addition to the changes you make in your diet, or by losing weight, or by taking steps to reduce inflammation and improve your sleep and stress levels, you can cut your diabetes risk by more than 25% by walking a total of three miles a day, equal to one hour of daily walking at a steady, moderate pace. Keep in mind, too, that these miles can be accumulated throughout the day, in increments as small as five or ten minutes. This is a goal that is easily achievable for most people, provided they build up to that level carefully, as prescribed later in this chapter.

Simply put, daily aerobic exercise is a **must** *if you have type 2 diabetes, prediabetes, or early insulin resistance.* If you have diabetes, exercise

Exercise: *Not for Type 2 Diabetics Only*

For those of you reading this book who have type 1 diabetes or know someone who does, I want to stress that exercise also has significant benefits for type 1 diabetics—in part because it increases HDL (good) cholesterol and improves blood vessel function, which can be critical in preventing the progression of diabetes-related cardiovascular complications. Our study of Joslin's Gold Medalists—people who have survived with type 1 diabetes for fifty years or more—shows that the amount of exercise they get correlates closely to protection against severe diabetic complications such as blindness, kidney failure, and nerve problems.

It's also worth noting that these and other positive changes induced by exercise will dramatically reduce your risk of cardiovascular disease, which is the major cause of death for people with type 1 and type 2 diabetes. In this regard, the HDL-boosting properties of exercise appear to have an especially protective effect in women with type 1 diabetes and, to a somewhat lesser extent, men. If women with type 1 diabetes can reach an HDL level of 60 or above, and if men with type 1 diabetes can achieve an HDL of 55 or above, their long-term survival rates improve significantly.

Exercise and Your Muscles: Getting the Fat Out

Although starting an exercise program can seem intimidating, it's important to realize that even a modest amount of exercise will help reduce the fat deposits in your muscles' cells within a very short amount of time. In one controlled study that compared diet and exercise to dieting alone, the subjects in the diet and exercise group expended an extra daily 70 calories over a period of two weeks. In case you're wondering, that's equivalent to a 190-pound person walking at a steady pace for ten minutes each day, or bicycling at a brisk tempo for eight minutes, or swimming the freestyle stroke for six and a half minutes—very doable, by anyone's standards.

By the end of that two weeks, the fat content inside the subjects' muscle cells had been reduced by almost 20%, the fat accumulation in their livers was decreased significantly, and their ability to metabolize infused glucose had risen by 57%!

will go a long way to lessening its impact. And if you have prediabetes or insulin resistance, following the exercise recommendations in this chapter can make the difference in terms of preventing your condition from progressing to type 2 diabetes.

Why Physical Activity Is Essential for Controlling Blood Glucose Levels

Although we're still unraveling exactly how physical movement affects our muscles, we already know some basic facts about why being physically active is one of the most effective things you can do to increase insulin sensitivity and prevent type 2 diabetes. For starters, experiments have shown that insulin resistance in the skeletal muscles—the muscles in our limbs, back, neck, head, and torso that we use for movement—accounts for about 90% of overall insulin resistance.

In other words, when your body is forced to overproduce insulin because you're not metabolizing glucose properly, it's due almost completely to the fact that your muscles have diminished insulin sensitivity and are no longer absorbing glucose from your bloodstream as efficiently as they should be. In addition, whenever you exercise for a few minutes or longer, your muscles become more sensitive to the effects of insulin—not only during exercise but up to forty-eight hours afterward. This means that every time you exercise, you'll absorb more glucose in your muscles for the next two days as the result of insulin's action, thereby reducing the amount of insulin your body has to pump out. This insulin-sensitizing effect appears to occur because of several factors detailed next.

Inside Joslin: Dr. King's Own Exercise Routine

When it comes to exercise, I am very careful to practice what I preach. It's my belief that once someone understands the powerful glucose-metabolizing effects of aerobic exercise and strength training—as I hope you will, after reading this chapter—then exercising will shift from being a chore to being an incredible opportunity to activate your muscles and normalize your metabolism.

My own routine, which I've followed for many years now, is much like the approach outlined in The Diabetes Reset—a mix of scheduled exercise, daily walking as a part of my normal activities, and a bit of recreational sports. The blend is different enough that whenever I get bored with one type of activity, I can rekindle my interest by switching to another.

I enjoy a regular workout every other day at my local health club, to capitalize on the forty-eight-hour boost in insulin sensitivity that exercising the muscles provides. This workout includes thirty minutes of running on a treadmill at a speed of ten to eleven minutes per mile (not very fast, but it does the job), followed by thirty minutes of strength training. In my strength routine, I work a variety of muscle groups in my arms, trunk, and legs, doing three sets of ten repetitions each on a dozen different weight-lifting machines, as well as sit-ups for my abdominal muscles.

On the days between my formal workouts, I do three sets of push-ups (fifty repetitions per set) and three sets of sit-ups (thirty to thirty-five repetitions per set). I also carry a pedometer at all times, and try to get in at least six thousand steps of walking every workday. I accomplish this by following some of the approaches suggested in this chapter: I try to park my car at least one block from wherever I'm heading and always walk the three to four flights of stairs in the parking garage near the Joslin Center, then walk up the five flights of stairs to my office. Because our building is just seven stories high, I also usually walk instead of taking the elevator when I'm going to meetings on other floors.

Finally, I make a point of playing tennis at least once a week for an hour and a half. I sometimes play singles, sometimes doubles, depending on who is available to play. Either way, my weekly tennis match is a great way to get my heart rate up, work all of the muscles in my body, and burn a few extra calories in the process. Plus, it's great fun!

When you exercise for an extended time, your muscles are actively burning glucose, which in turn reduces the levels of glycogen—the stored form of glucose—in your muscle tissues. Glycogen levels appear to be directly related to insulin sensitivity: The lower they are, the more sensitive your muscles are to insulin. This also means that the longer you work out (and the more glycogen you metabolize), the more you'll temporarily reduce your insulin resistance.

Because your muscles run on a mix of fuels, including both glucose and fatty acids, exercise also metabolizes the fat deposits in your muscles, which also appears to be directly related to improved insulin sensitivity. One study found that in people who are obese, a single exercise session reduced the amount of fat inside the muscles. Again, the longer you exercise, the more fatty acids your muscles will metabolize.

Whenever you exercise your muscles, you are also activating certain enzymes and proteins that mimic what insulin does but work *independently* of insulin to help your muscles absorb glucose from the bloodstream. One key biochemical in this process is AMP-activated protein kinase (AMPK), a protein that Dr. Goodyear and her colleagues have been studying intensively and is activated by muscle contractions. Scientists have shown that these exercise-related glucose uptake mechanisms continue to function even when someone has insulin resistance and that their effects last for a couple of hours after exercising. So even if your body is highly insulin resistant, exercise can still temporarily normalize your muscles' ability to absorb blood glucose through an entirely separate process.

Insulin resistance in the skeletal muscles also appears to be linked to impaired function of the mitochondria—the microscopic "energy factories" in the muscle cells that are responsible for converting oxygen, glucose, amino acids, and fatty acids into the energy that powers your muscles' contractions. When these tiny factories are not metabolizing fuel as well as they should, they produce free radicals—ionized oxygen particles that have also been found to interfere with insulin signaling. In Strategy Chapter 8, I'll discuss these particles and how to neutralize them at greater length. Joslin researchers have found that this impairment appears to be related to decreased levels of an enzyme called Sirt3. People with type 2 diabetes have just half the amount of this enzyme inside their mitochondria as nondiabetics. Exercise, on the other hand, has been shown to markedly increase Sirt3 activity in the skeletal muscles.

In addition, when you're exercising you are encouraging fat loss because exercise also triggers fat stores to release fatty acids as backup fuel. Unlike the raised levels of FFA in a resting state, which accumulate in the muscles, fatty acids released during exercise are taken into the muscles and oxidized for energy.

Over the long term, regular aerobic exercise also increases both the sheer number and the functional ability of the mitochondria in the muscles being exercised, enabling them to produce much more energy from oxygen mixed with glucose and fats, and thereby allowing the muscles to function at a high level longer. This increase in mitochondrial activity is the primary reason endurance increases through aerobic training. All other exercise-related enhancements, including increases in your muscles' ability to store energy, the growth of additional capillaries (tiny blood vessels) in your exercising muscles, your heart's ability to pump more blood with each contraction, and improvements in your body's ability to dissipate heat, are adaptations designed to service the increased activity of your muscles' mitochondria. Besides making it easier to exercise for a sustained period of time, this increase in mitochondrial function also further enhances your muscles' ability to metabolize glucose and fats both during exercise and at rest.

Finally, people who take up regular physical activity as part of

The Forty-Eight-Hour Effect

Laboratory experiments have determined that the insulin-sensitizing effects of exercise last for forty-eight hours. For this reason, I recommend that you never let more than two days go by without putting in a concerted session of physical activity. This effect also means that you will see improvements in insulin resistance even if you exercise only every other day. As noted elsewhere in this chapter, however, you will see significantly more results if you exercise six or seven days a week at the levels suggested in the Diabetes Reset exercise strategy.

a weight-loss program generally find it easier to lose weight and keep it off compared to those who try to lose weight through dieting alone—in part by raising the metabolic rate, which tends to drop when you begin cutting your intake of calories. And as we've already seen, losing weight is one of the most important things you can do to help reverse diabetes and prediabetes, both by reducing the overall inflammation that excess weight can cause and by helping to eliminate the fat deposits in your muscles that lead to insulin resistance.

The powerful benefits that exercise brings are the reason why physical activity has been a core part of Joslin's treatment approach to diabetes from the very beginning. For many years, we were one of the only diabetes centers in the U.S. to maintain a gym and employ full-time exercise physiologists. It also explains why Dr. Goodyear and I both exercise regularly: She does a ninety-minute swimming workout three mornings a week as well as three weekly strength training workouts, while I do a mix of different activities. (See box on page 111: Inside Joslin: Dr. King's Own Exercise Routine.)

First Step: Get Your Doctor's Go-Ahead

If you've been relatively inactive in recent years, your first step before beginning your new exercise program should be a visit to your regular doctor. In setting up the appointment, explain that you're planning to start a new routine of daily physical activity and that you want a thorough exam first to make sure there aren't any health concerns you need to be aware of in addition to your blood glucose issues. Your doctor's exam should include a thorough evaluation of your cardiovascular health, which will entail complete blood tests and a check of your heart and lung function and blood pressure. Your doctor may also recommend a stress test, in which you walk on a treadmill or ride an exercise bike while an EKG is used to monitor your heart's electrical activity. This test is used to diagnose any significant blockages in your coronary arteries. Be aware, however, that passing a stress test does not mean your arteries are completely clear—just that any blockages that might be present aren't large enough to cause symptoms during the test.

Once you have the results of your exam, outline the specific exercise program you're planning to embark on and make sure you get your doctor's green light to proceed.

In addition to these "official" workouts, both of us—like many other members of the Joslin staff—spend as much time moving about during the day as possible, strolling the halls to confer with colleagues instead of phoning, using the stairwells instead of the elevators, and generally trying to minimize the time we spend sitting in office chairs or at the wheel of a car.

All this daily movement speaks to the point made by Dr. Goodyear at the start of this chapter: Although there is considerable value in regular exercise sessions, your body benefits from *any* kind of physical activity, even if it's just a few minutes spent walking up the staircase of your office building or bicycling over to your neighbor's house. Every movement, from hefting a bag of groceries to raking leaves, helps stimulate your muscles' diabetes-fighting properties, while every moment spent sitting or lying down is an opportunity for insulin resistance to continue advancing. That's why it's important to move as much as possible *all* the time—not just during scheduled exercise sessions.

In the pages that follow, I'll lay out some specific recommendations on how to incorporate more exercise into your life. But if there's one thing you take away from this chapter, I hope it's that you'll start thinking about *sitting less and moving more* every waking moment of the day. Each minute you spend out of a chair and on your feet is a minute that will help you improve the insulin sensitivity of your muscles, start reversing the progression of prediabetes and type 2 diabetes, and prevent the diabetes-related complications that both type 1 and type 2 diabetes can cause.

Putting Your Own Exercise Plan into Action

When it comes to reversing insulin resistance, the more you move your body's muscles, the better. Remember, every muscle contraction brings diabetes-fighting benefits. At the same time, with all the focus on "working out" and target heart rates and going to the gym, the first and most important way to become more active is to begin adding more aerobic activity into your daily life. The Diabetes Reset aerobic exercise plan is based on several key principles:

Walking Your Way to Better Health

When planning your new aerobic lifestyle, you can choose from a wide range of activities, including bicycling, running, swimming, aerobics classes, or working out on aerobic exercise devices such as stationary bikes and elliptical trainers at a local health club. In general, however, I recommend to everyone that they begin with a plan to incorporate more walking into their daily life. Walking has a number of advantages that make it the perfect foundation for a program of daily physical activity:

• It can be done virtually anywhere, in any type of weather.

• It requires no equipment beyond a good pair of walking shoes.

• It is a very low-impact activity, which means it carries minimal injury risk and can be done even by people with musculoskeletal conditions such as arthritis or chronic back pain.

• It can easily be done in groups and also allows conversation while exercising—both critical points because people exercise much more consistently when they can make it part of a social gathering.

• Making sure you're getting at least five thousand steps of casual, "incidental" walking each day, in the course of your normal daily activities.

• Taking frequent breaks from sitting throughout the day, even if this means simply getting up and walking a few steps to the water cooler at work or your kitchen at home.

• Getting at least twenty-five minutes per day (equivalent to 2,500 steps) of additional brisk walking or other moderate-intensity aerobic activity on six days out of each week, with one rest day. This amount of activity, which adds up to a total of 150 minutes of moderate-intensity aerobic exercise per week, represents Level I in the Diabetes Reset aerobics program.

• If you want to reduce your diabetes risk and improve your glucose control even more, then I recommend increasing the amount of moderate-intensity aerobic activity you do each day (above and beyond your five thousand steps of incidental walking) to fifty minutes—the equivalent of another five thousand steps of brisk walking. This amount of activity, which adds up to a total of three hundred minutes of moderate-intensity aerobic exercise per week, represents Level II in the Diabetes Reset aerobics program.

Finding Your "Walking Windows"

L ately, exercise experts have been playing close attention to the important health benefits of daily physical movement outside formal exercise sessions. Simply standing up, for example, increases your energy expenditure by 25% compared to sitting, while a slow 1-mph walking pace will burn more than half the calories that you'll expend at a brisk, 3-mph walking pace—meaning that a leisurely hour-long stroll actually burns about as much calories as a thirty-minute power walk.

How Much Should You Exercise Each Day?

T he research indicates that when it comes to improving your insulin sensitivity and glucose metabolism, there are essentially two levels of daily exercise you can aim for:

- *Level I: Five thousand incidental steps of walking per day, plus twenty-five hundred steps (another twenty-five minutes) of intentional brisk walking per day or twenty-five minutes of another aerobic activity done at moderate intensity (10 to 13 on the Perceived Exertion scale; see sidebar on page 120).* This level will reduce your risk of developing type 2 diabetes by about 20% if you have prediabetes, independent of any other measures you take, and has also been shown to lower hemoglobin A1C levels in people with type 2 diabetes by slightly more than .4, on average.

- *Level II: Five thousand incidental steps a day, plus five thousand steps (fifty minutes) of intentional brisk walking per day or fifty minutes of another aerobic activity done at moderate intensity (10 to 13 on the Perceived Exertion scale).* This is a good amount of exercise, but if you can manage it, you will see very positive results. If you have prediabetes and can achieve this level of activity or its equivalent, you will cut your type 2 diabetes risk almost in half, independent of any other measures you take. If you already have type 2 diabetes, this amount of exercise has been shown to reduce A1C levels by 1.1, on average.

Researchers have found that people can usually find ways to take five thousand steps a day in their ordinary activities—at work, traveling from place to place, and doing basic chores around their home—if they make a habit of finding opportunities to engage in this type of "incidental" walking. To help you do this, I advise purchasing a good, inexpensive pedometer. A very reliable model can generally be obtained for $30 or less. (See box: Walk This Way: Leading Pedometers for $30 and Less.) Then aim to take five thousand steps in the course of your normal activities each day.

Once you start looking for opportunities in your daily routine to slip in a few minutes of walking, you'll find that these "walking windows" are actually quite plentiful. In addition to ones you've already heard about—parking a block from where you're heading or on a higher level in the parking garage and walking the rest of the way, getting off the subway or bus a stop early, taking the stairs instead of the elevator, and walking to a coworker's workspace instead of emailing or phoning—here are a few you may not have thought of:

- Place a treadmill or exercise bike in front of your TV and exercise for the duration of a favorite show.

- Install a "walking desk"—a small treadmill and standing desk—in your workplace.

- Suggest to your work colleagues that you hold "walking meetings" instead of sitting around a conference table.

- In cold or inclement weather, get creative: Find a nearby mall, school, or gym where you can set up an indoor walking circuit.

The Importance of Moderate-Intensity Aerobic Exercise

Although incidental walking and breaks from sitting are important, research shows that if you want to significantly reduce your risk for type 2 diabetes and improve your glucose control, you also have to engage in some sort of higher-intensity aerobic exercise most

Walk This Way: Leading Pedometers for $30 and Less

Pedometers have come a long way in recent years. Today's brands are lightweight and versatile, and tend to be highly accurate at normal walking speeds. Here are several manufacturers that offer well-regarded products for under $30.

- *Omron.* The pedometers made by this medical device manufacturer consistently top the ratings lists and have also been used in clinical trials.

- *Yamax.* Another consistently well-rated manufacturer whose products are widely used in clinical trials.

Yamax models are also sold under the Accusplit brand name.

- *Bodytronics.* This company's ProStep Dual Step Counter, available for less than $20, has a dual counter system that tracks both daily and cumulative step totals.

- *Your favorite smartphone.* Many smartphones have free pedometer apps available, including the Apple iPhone, Android-powered phones such as the Samsung Galaxy, and BlackBerry phones.

days of every week. This could be brisk walking at a steady pace or any other aerobic exercise involving large muscle groups, such as cycling, swimming, jogging, aerobic dance, cross-country skiing, rowing, riding a stationary bike, or using an elliptical trainer or stair-climber at a health club.

Research also indicates that the point where significant benefits for glucose control occur is when you do 150 minutes of this type of moderate-intensity exercise per week—the equivalent of 25 minutes of exercise, six days per week. Achieving this amount of aerobic activity, which I call Aerobic Exercise Level I, is a key goal of the Diabetes Reset Plan. If you can do twice this amount—50 minutes a day, six days a week, for a weekly total of 300 minutes—you'll benefit even more, a fact clearly borne out by studies that have followed individuals at risk for type 2 diabetes over time. By engaging in this level of activity, which I call Aerobic Exercise Level II, you cut your statistical risk of developing type 2 diabetes in half—and that's *without* taking into account your other Diabetes Reset strategies!

Note, by the way, that I'm talking about *total* daily exercise here. You don't have to do all of this exercise in a single session to get its full benefits. In fact, some intriguing research was recently published suggesting that in terms of improved insulin sensitivity, you may actually get better results by breaking up your daily aerobic exercise into shorter sessions throughout the day—doing three brisk ten-minute walks, for example, rather than a single thirty-minute walk.

Using "Perceived Exertion" to Guide Your Workouts

Although some people choose to wear heart monitors to gauge exactly how hard they're working out, that isn't really necessary. Research shows that people can pinpoint their level of effort very accurately by using the Borg Scale of Perceived Exertion. This scale, developed by Swedish physiologist Gunnar Borg, goes from 6 to 20—the reason being that when you multiply the various levels of exertion on the scale by 10, they correspond roughly to the heart rate produced in the average healthy adult during exercise. A level of 6, for example, would produce essentially a resting heart rate of 60 beats per minute, whereas an exertion level of 12 would produce a heart rate of 120 beats per minute.

When doing aerobic exercise, to get maximal benefits while avoiding overexertion, you should be in the 9 to 11 range of this scale for the first five minutes or so as you're warming up your muscles and connective tissue and in the 10 to 13 range for the rest of your activity session. Strength training should generally involve an effort in the 15 to 17 range.

THE BORG SCALE: HOW HARD DOES YOUR EFFORT FEEL RIGHT NOW?	
6	
7	Very, very light
8	
9	Very light
10	
11	Fairly light
12	
13	Somewhat hard
14	
15	Hard
16	
17	Very hard
18	
19	Very, very hard
20	

Here's another rule of thumb that will help you know you're at 13 or less on the Borg scale: Whenever you are doing an aerobic activity, you should always be exercising at a "talking" pace—meaning that you're never so short of breath that you can't carry on a conversation with your walking partner.

What kind of exercise should you do? Our experience at Joslin working with patients from many different backgrounds has shown that the most important aspect of any exercise program is that it *works for that individual.* To design a workout plan that is both practical and enjoyable, start with the following guidelines.

- **Choose an activity you already know how to do.** Pick a continuous, familiar activity such as walking, swimming, cycling, dancing (aerobic or ballroom), or working out on a stationary bike, elliptical trainer, rowing machine, or stair-climber that is familiar and that you have ready access to. I suggest avoiding high-impact activities like running because these activities are hard on your knees, hips, and other joints, as well as very low-intensity activities like yoga and tai chi, which don't work the muscles enough to be an effective primary activity for reducing insulin resistance (although they can certainly make a fine add-on activity, of course).

- **If possible, pick a regular time of day to exercise that fits into your schedule well.** The best time to exercise is *anytime you can do it*: before or after work, during your lunch break, before you go to bed—it really doesn't matter.

- **Make specific appointments for each workout.** Use your computer or smartphone's calendar, or buy a monthly wall calendar—one with good-sized boxes for each day so that you have plenty of writing room—and jot down each appointment. Example: "Strength training at 5:30 p.m." on Wednesday and Friday of a given week or "30 minutes of swimming—7:00 a.m." on your scheduled pool days.

- **Begin slowly.** Start with ten-minute exercise sessions, then increase the length of your workouts by five minutes each week until you're exercising for thirty minutes at a time.

- **Aim for at least 150 minutes of aerobic exercise per week.** A number of large-scale studies have found that this amount of exercise—which can be achieved by doing thirty minutes of exercise per day for at least five days each week—is optimal for improving insulin sensitivity and lowering type 2 diabetes risk.

- **Take at least one "rest day" per week.** Research has also shown that people who exercise seven days a week tend to suffer overuse injuries at a much higher rate than those who forego a formal workout for at least one day per week. I'm not saying that you should lie around in a hammock on your rest days—but taking one or two days off from your formal workout routine each week is clearly beneficial in the long run. Just don't take off two days in a row because the insulin-enhancing benefits of exercise fade after forty-eight hours.

- **Consider joining an exercise group or recruiting a regular exercise partner.** Studies have shown that the people who stick to their programs tend to be those who arrange to meet regularly with other exercisers in some formalized way. (See box on page 125: Inside Joslin: A Group Walk for Health.) You don't have to exercise with others every day—but try to get together at least once a week: Join a walking, running, or cycling club that has regular group sessions, agree to meet with one or more friends at a regular time each week for a group workout, or find a way to exercise with your spouse on a weekly basis. (Ballroom dancing and cycling are both great activities for couples.)

Get Serious with Strength Training: Adding Resistance Exercise to Your Routine

Research has shown conclusively that you can reduce insulin resistance and improve your glucose metabolism even more if you supplement your aerobic exercise with regular sessions of resistance training—also known as strength training—in which you work against a fairly heavy resistance, using thick resistance bands, handheld weights, or weight machines designed to strengthen specific muscle groups. A review of thirteen randomized controlled trials that was published in 2010, for example, found that resistance training significantly lowered average blood glucose levels in people with prediabetes or type 2 diabetes.

In part, this is due to the fact that resistance training increases overall muscle mass by enlarging the size of individual muscle fibers. And

If You Take Insulin Medication, Read This Before Exercising

The quick insulin-sensitivity boost that you get from exercise is generally a good thing. If you take insulin medication for type 1 or type 2 diabetes, however, you need to take extra precautions when you're exercising—otherwise, your extra insulin sensitivity could combine with your insulin medication to drive your blood glucose levels too low, causing you to become hypoglycemic. To help avoid this, never inject insulin into your arm and leg if you plan to exercise within the next several hours—the extra blood flow through your limbs can cause the insulin to take effect too quickly. Instead, inject it into your abdomen, where it will be absorbed more slowly. In addition, when starting your new exercise routine, I recommend taking along a high-carbohydrate snack while you work out, in case you suffer a drop in glucose levels, and checking your blood glucose midway through your workout and again right after you finish to gauge how your glucose levels are being affected by exercise.

because the muscles are where 90% of insulin-related glucose uptake takes place, this gives insulin more tissue to work with, so to speak. An analysis of thirteen thousand adult subjects, based on the U.S. government's third National Health and Nutrition Examination Survey (NHANES III) and published in 2011, divided survey participants into four quartiles, depending on how much muscle mass they had as a percentage of their total body weight. The researchers found that the greater the subjects' muscle mass, the lower their levels of insulin resistance and average blood glucose levels were, and the less likely they were to have prediabetes or diabetes.

This effect has added importance for people who already have type 2 diabetes because they tend to lose muscle mass faster than others as they get older, due to reduced nerve stimulation of muscle fibers. But increased muscle mass isn't the only story: Other researchers have found that resistance training also improves glucose uptake in the muscles by stimulating positive chemical changes in the muscle fibers that are different from the positive changes induced by aerobic exercise.

Strength training has other benefits for people with diabetes or pre-diabetes, too. By increasing muscle mass, it boosts base metabolic rate and aids in weight loss. In addition, strength training, especially of the leg and trunk muscles, helps improve balance and reduces the likelihood of dangerous falls—something individuals with type 2 diabetes are at increased risk for due to nerve damage.

Designing Your Own Strength Training Routine

An effective strength training workout generally consists of eight to ten exercises, each of which work a different muscle group to a point of near-fatigue over a period of about two minutes. This training approach taxes the short-term anaerobic (non-oxygen-related) energy system in the muscles, which causes the fiber muscles to become larger and stronger—as opposed to aerobic (oxygen-related) exercise, which builds endurance rather than size and strength. You can do strength training with various types of resistance, including resistance tubing or bands (thick lengths of elastic that you can push against with your limbs), dumbbells or barbells (weights that you can pick up and hold in your hands), or weight machines like those made by Nautilus or Cybex, which are typically found in health clubs or gyms (though multipurpose machines are also sold for home use).

RESISTANCE EXERCISE OPTIONS: PROS AND CONS

- **Resistance tubing.** At Joslin, we use a resistance tubing exercise routine with many of our patients. Resistance tubing is a length of rubberlike hose with handles for each hand. It can be easily used at home by looping the tubing around your foot or torso, doors, posts, or heavy furniture. (Simple lengths of rubberlike material such as Therabands can also be adapted for these exercises, though you'll need to make knotted loops out of them or create knotted handles at the ends of them to avoid having to grip them between your fingers as you exercise.) They are also inexpensive—you can purchase them online from a wide range of manufacturers starting at around $10 per individual piece (just type in "resistance band" or "resistance tubing" in your Internet search engine)—and they are completely portable, with a single band or tube length easily fitting into a pants or coat pocket. They come in varying levels of resistance as well, allowing you to increase resistance as you build more strength in a given muscle group.

• **Dumbbells**. Dumbbells are also fairly inexpensive and can be used and stored easily at home. They can be more challenging to manipulate than resistance tubing or resistance bands, however, and moving up in resistance will require adding plates to an adjustable dumbbell or buying a series of dumbbells of varying weights. That said, working out with dumbbells is a very effective way to improve

Inside Joslin: A Group Walk for Health

Turning aerobic exercise into a social event is one of the best ways to ensure that you get regular exercise. At Joslin, our Asian American Diabetes Initiative launched a regular group walking program for Asian Americans in the Boston area. Many Asian Americans already do tai chi on a regular basis—but although tai chi is good for a number of things, including balance, flexibility, and circulation, it doesn't really work the skeletal muscles enough to improve their glucose-burning ability. So we invited members of the community to meet weekly at the Boston Commons for a half hour or more of brisk walking. We had a small turnout for the first session or two, but once word spread about how energizing and enjoyable these group workouts were, our numbers quickly hit the one hundred mark. We're currently embarking on a clinical trial that will utilize this program to investigate how walking as a group compares with exercising alone in terms of helping individuals maintain a healthy program of physical activity.

What to Do

Many communities have similar group walking programs or clubs that meet in local parks or at indoor shopping malls or civic centers in cold or inclement weather. To find a program near you, contact your local YM/YWCA or visit the website of the American Volkssport Association, which has contact information for hundreds of clubs across the U.S. If you're interested in finding a running club in your area (which typically welcomes walkers, as well), visit the Road Runners Club of America website and click the Find a Running Club tab for a state-by-state guide to the thousands of running organizations throughout the nation.

muscular strength and body mass for the targeted muscle group while also building the peripheral muscle control required to hold and manipulate the weight.

- **Weight machines.** These are probably the most effective way to build strength and muscle mass in a variety of muscle groups. Because you are pushing the resistance bar of these machines along a fixed track, they can be used easily and safely even by beginners, and the typical "pin" design of these machines allows you to easily increase or decrease the amount of weight you're using. A good gym or club will also offer a wide range of such machines, enabling you to work all of the body's different muscle groups. The main downside of these machines is that you generally need to have access to a gym or health club to take advantage of them—which can be costly and also time-consuming. That said, if there is a convenient, reasonably priced health club near you that offers a good range of weight machines, you may want to consider getting a membership.

- **Home weight machines.** These machines typically feature a dozen or so different strength training exercises in one multipurpose unit. Many people have had success with these, but they have drawbacks as well, over and above their cost. Although they can be fairly compact, they still require a significant amount of floor space, and they are also generally not quite as effective or user-friendly as the high-end weight machines in health clubs.

Principles of Strength Training

When doing a strength training workout, set aside at least a half hour, which will give you time to do eight to ten exercises working various muscle groups.

- Try to alternate lower body and upper body exercises, moving from the larger muscle groups to the smaller muscle groups.

- Each exercise should involve one or more "sets" of ten to fifteen repetitions, using enough resistance so that the last repetition feels fairly hard. If you finish a set and you feel like you could have done several more repetitions, the weight is too light. If you can't do ten repetitions, then the weight is too heavy.

- Don't rush your repetitions: Move in a steady, fluid motion, breathing out as you push against the weight and inhaling as you return to the starting position.

- For best results, do at least two resistance workouts each week, always taking at least forty-eight hours between training sessions to let your muscle tissue recover.

Important: If you have diabetes-related eye problems, consult with your physician before doing any of the exercise routines that follow. Strength training can cause dangerous pressure to build up inside the eyes, leading to damage in susceptible individuals.

Strength Training Routine 1: The Joslin Resistance Tubing Routine

- **Equipment**: One or more pieces of resistance tubing of varying resistance levels.

- **Instructions***:* Do three sets of each of the following exercises. Each set should consist of ten to fifteen repetitions of a given movement. If the last repetition feels easy, move up to a piece of tubing with more resistance.

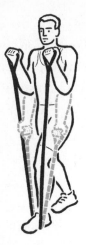

EXERCISE 1: STANDING CURL
MUSCLES WORKED: BICEPS

Stand with one foot in front of the other as if you're striding forward. Anchor the tubing under your front foot, then stand holding the handles of the tubing with palms facing upward. Curl your arms up so your fists are almost touching your shoulders, exhaling as you do, then slowly return to the starting position.

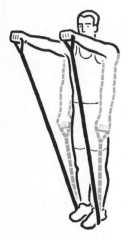

EXERCISE 2: ALTERNATE ARM RAISE
MUSCLES WORKED: SHOULDERS AND UPPER BACK

Stand with your feet close together and anchor the tubing under both feet. Hold the handles of the tubing with palms facing down, then raise one arm in front of you until it is parallel to the floor, exhaling as you do. Lower slowly, then repeat with the alternate arm.

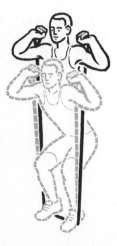

EXERCISE 3: SQUAT
MUSCLES WORKED: QUADRICEPS, HAMSTRINGS, BUTTOCKS, AND BACK

Stand with your feet at shoulder width and anchor the tubing under both feet. Hold the handles of the tubing at shoulder height with palms facing upward. Squat down, inhaling as you do and keeping your back straight. Then exhale as you slowly return to standing, working against the resistance.

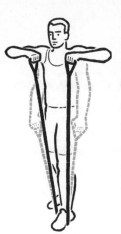

EXERCISE 4: UPRIGHT ROW
MUSCLES WORKED: SHOULDER AND UPPER BACK

Stand with one foot in front of the other as if you're striding forward. Anchor the tubing under your front foot, then stand holding the tubing with palms facing downward. Raise both hands slowly toward your chin, pointing your elbows outward and exhaling as you do, then slowly return to the starting position.

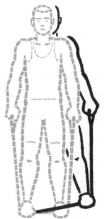

EXERCISE 5: WALKING SIDE TO SIDE
MUSCLES WORKED: OUTER THIGHS, BUTTOCKS, AND ABDOMINAL MUSCLES

Stand with your feet at shoulder width and anchor tubing under both feet. Holding the handles with your hands at your sides, walk ten to fifteen steps to your right, and then ten to fifteen steps to your left.

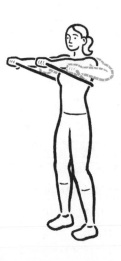

EXERCISE 6: STANDING CHEST PRESS
MUSCLES WORKED: PECTORALS IN FRONT OF CHEST

Loop the resistance tubing around a post or other stationary object at chest height, then stand facing the opposite direction. (Alternately, you can loop the tubing around your back and grasp the tubing somewhere above each handle to shorten its effective length.) Start with the handles (or area of the tubing you are gripping) close to your body with your elbows bent and pulled back. Extend your arms out straight, exhaling as you do, then slowly return to the starting position.

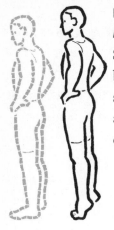

EXERCISE 7: HEEL RAISE
MUSCLES WORKED: CALVES

Standing with your hand on your hips, rise up on the balls of your feet, exhaling as you do, then return slowly to the starting position. (Alternatively, you can anchor the tubing under your feet and hold the handles near your shoulders to increase the resistance.)

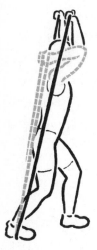

EXERCISE 8: STANDING OVERHEAD PRESS
MUSCLES WORKED: TRICEPS

Stand with one foot in front of the other as if you're striding forward. Anchor the tubing under your back foot, then hold both handles behind your head with your thumbs pointing downward. Straighten your arms so they extend up above your head, rotating your palms forward and exhaling as you do, then slowly return to the starting position.

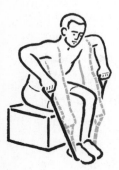

EXERCISE 9: SITTING SHOULDER ROW WITH TRUNK FLEXION
MUSCLES WORKED: MIDDLE BACK

Sit on a bench or hard chair with your feet together and the tubing anchored beneath both feet. Lean slightly forward, holding both handles with your palms facing down. Pull your elbows back and upward, squeezing your shoulder blades together and exhaling as you do, then slowly return to the starting position.

Strength Workout 2: Dumbbell Routine

- **Equipment:** A set of dumbbells of varying weights or a pair of adjustable dumbbells.

- **Instructions:** Do one to two sets of each of the following exercises. A set consists of ten to fifteen repetitions of a given movement. Once the last repetition starts feeling easy for a given exercise, move up to a slightly heavier weight.

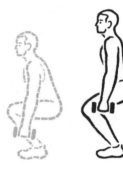

EXERCISE 1: SQUAT
MUSCLES WORKED: QUADRICEPS, HAMSTRING, BUTTOCKS, AND BACK
Stand with your feet flat on the floor, shoulder's width apart. Hold both dumbbells at your side with arms extended, then slowly lower your hips until your thighs are parallel to the floor. Keeping your back straight, rise to the standing position, exhaling as you do.

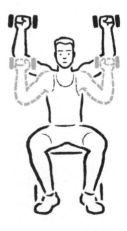

EXERCISE 2: SHOULDER PRESS
MUSCLES WORKED: SHOULDERS, UPPER BACK, AND TRICEPS
Sit upright on the edge of a bench or chair, holding a dumbbell in each hand. Bring the weights to shoulder level with your palms facing away from your body. Next, press both dumbbells directly over your head, moving them toward each other so that at the top of the movement they're gently touching, exhaling as you do. Then slowly lower the dumbbells back to the starting position.

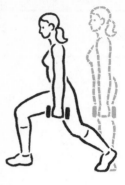

EXERCISE 3: LUNGE
MUSCLES WORKED: QUADRICEPS, CALVES, HAMSTRINGS, AND BUTTOCKS

Stand holding both dumbbells with your arms at your sides. Take a long step forward with one foot, so that your lead knee is directly over your ankle. Next, bend your rear leg so that your knee approaches the floor. Then push off with your front foot and return to the starting position, exhaling as you do. Do ten to fifteen repetitions, then switch sides and repeat.

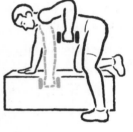

EXERCISE 4: DUMBBELL ROW
MUSCLES WORKED: BACK, SHOULDERS, BICEPS, AND FOREARMS

Place your right hand and knee on a flat bench so that your back is horizontal. Hold a dumbbell in your left hand and let it hang downward with your arm extended. Keeping your elbow close to your body, pull the dumbbell up toward your chest, exhaling as you do, then slowly lower the dumbbell back to the starting position. Do ten to fifteen repetitions, then switch sides and repeat.

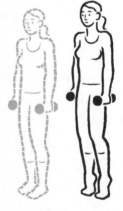

EXERCISE 5: HEEL RAISE
MUSCLES WORKED: CALVES

Stand with your feet at shoulder width. Holding a dumbbell in each hand, rise up on the balls of your feet, exhaling as you do, then slowly return to the starting position.

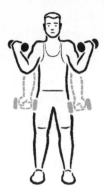

EXERCISE 6: CURL

MUSCLES WORKED: BICEPS

Stand with your feet slightly apart or sit upright on the edge of a flat bench or chair. Holding a dumbbell in each hand, extend your arms downward with your palms facing forward. Keeping your back straight, lift both dumbbells up toward your shoulders, exhaling as you do, then slowly lower the dumbbells back to the starting position.

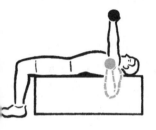

EXERCISE 7: CHEST PRESS

MUSCLES WORKED: CHEST, SHOULDERS, AND TRICEPS

Lie faceup on a bench or the floor, with knees bent and feet flat on the ground. Hold a dumbbell in each hand, palms facing upward, and bring them to shoulder level with your elbows pointing out to the sides. Next, extend both arms fully to raise the dumbbells directly over your chest, exhaling as you do, then slowly lower the dumbbells back to the starting position.

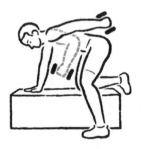

EXERCISE 8: TRICEPS EXTENSION

MUSCLES WORKED: TRICEPS IN BACK OF UPPER ARMS

Holding a dumbbell in your left hand, place your right hand and knee on a bench. With the palm of your left hand facing in, bend your left arm so that the dumbbell is next to your hip. Keeping your left shoulder stationary, extend your left arm straight behind you, exhaling as you do, then slowly return to the starting position. Do ten to fifteen repetitions, then switch sides and repeat.

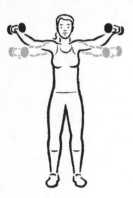

EXERCISE 9: SHOULDER RAISE

MUSCLES WORKED: OUTER SHOULDERS

Stand with your feet apart. Hold both dumbbells at your sides with your elbows bent. Keeping your elbows bent and your palms facing downward, raise the dumbbells until they are slightly higher than shoulder level, exhaling as you do, then slowly return to the starting position.

Strength Training Workout 3: Weight Machine Routine

- **Equipment**: A gym or health club fully equipped with multiple weight-lifting machines, or a multistation home weight machine.

- **Instructions**: Do one to two sets of each of the following exercises. A set consists of ten to fifteen repetitions of a given movement. Once the last repetition starts feeling easy for a given exercise, move up to a slightly heavier weight. If you are at a health club or gym and are using one of these machines for the first time, ask one of the employees to show you the proper form and help you select a starting weight.

EXERCISE 1: LEG PRESS MACHINE

MUSCLES WORKED: QUADRICEPS, BUTTOCKS, AND CALVES

EXERCISE 2: SHOULDER PRESS MACHINE

MUSCLES WORKED: SHOULDERS, UPPER BACK, AND TRICEPS

EXERCISE 3: LEG EXTENSION MACHINE

MUSCLES WORKED: QUADRICEPS

EXERCISE 4: CHEST PRESS MACHINE

MUSCLES WORKED: CHEST, SHOULDERS, AND TRICEPS

EXERCISE 5: LEG CURL MACHINE

MUSCLES WORKED: HAMSTRINGS

EXERCISE 6: TRICEPS MACHINE
MUSCLES WORKED: TRICEPS

EXERCISE 7: CALF RAISE
MUSCLES WORKED: CALVES

EXERCISE 8: ARM CURL MACHINE
MUSCLES WORKED: BICEPS

EXERCISE 9: LAT PULLDOWN MACHINE
MUSCLES WORKED: MIDDLE BACK

Five Stretches for Better Performance

As we age, certain muscle groups tend to shorten somewhat. Gently stretching these muscles on a daily basis will help you keep your leg, hip, and torso muscles in balance, reducing your chances of an overuse injury and allowing you to maintain a more fluid movement as you exercise. The following easy stretches take only a few minutes. They require no equipment whatsoever and can be done anywhere.

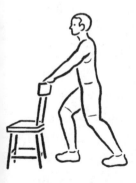

CALF AND ACHILLES STRETCH

Stand comfortably with your hands on your hips or hold the back of a chair for balance. Step backward with one foot so that your toes are a short distance behind the opposite heel. Keeping your feet flat on the floor, bend both knees slightly as you shift your weight onto your rear leg. Bend your knees farther to sink slowly downward until you feel a gentle stretching sensation along the back of the lower leg and heel of your rear leg. Hold for fifteen to thirty seconds, breathing slowly and deeply, then change legs and repeat.

HAMSTRING STRETCH

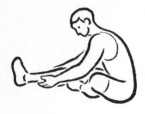

Sit on the floor with one leg stretched in front of you and the other leg bent so that the bottom of your foot rests against the inside of your straight leg. Slowly lower your forehead toward the knee of your extended leg until you feel a gentle stretch down the back of your thigh. Hold for fifteen to thirty seconds, breathing slowly and deeply, then change legs and repeat.

LOWER BACK STRETCH

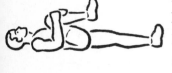

Lying on your back, grasp one knee with both hands and pull it as closely to your chest as you can. Breathe in deeply then exhale, relaxing as you do, and pull the knee toward your chest again. Hold for ten to fifteen seconds, then return to the starting position. Do this several times, then switch legs and repeat.

CHEST STRETCH

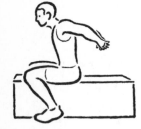

Standing comfortably or sitting on a bench, inter-lace your fingers behind your back with your arms extended straight back and your palms facing your back. Lift your hands up to the ceiling until you feel a gentle stretching sensation in the front of your chest. Keeping your neck relaxed, hold for fifteen to thirty seconds, breathing slowly and deeply.

HIP STRETCH

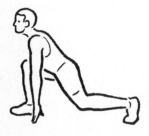

With one knee resting on the floor, step forward with your other leg so that your knee is directly above your ankle. Slowly lower the hip of your rear leg to the ground until you feel a gentle stretching sensation in the front of that hip. Hold for ten to fif-teen seconds then return to the starting position. Do this several times, then switch legs and repeat.

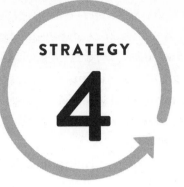

ACTIVATE YOUR CALORIE-BURNING BROWN FAT— IT'S EASIER THAN YOU THINK

Brown fat is a special type of body fat, found in small amounts in most (and perhaps all) people, that burns calories at a very high rate when activated by cold temperatures or other triggers—as much as several hundred calories a day. Some scientists believe that if we could all learn to activate our brown fat on a regular basis—following the approaches outlined in this chapter—it could help put an end to America's obesity epidemic.

"**W**ith brown fat you have a tissue that, just a few years ago, wasn't thought to exist functionally in adult humans. How often do you get a moment in your career where you're part of a group that discovers a new functional organ in humans? It just doesn't happen!"

When Aaron Cypess, M.D., Ph.D., talks about brown fat, you can sense his excitement. Several years ago, Dr. Cypess teamed up with other Joslin colleagues, including pioneering diabetes researcher Dr. C. Ronald Kahn, to publish an article that created waves around the world. In the article, which appeared in the *New England Journal of Medicine* in the spring of 2009, Drs. Cypess and Kahn reported they had reviewed PET-CT scans of nearly two thousand adults, looking for pockets of fat tissue that were metabolizing unusually high amounts of glucose—a hallmark of active brown fat. They found observable brown fat deposits in about 7% of the women and 3% of the men who had been scanned, mostly in their necks and the front of their chests.

Why was this such a paradigm-shattering publication? First, because up until then, it had been assumed that only babies and children had functioning brown fat (or, as scientists like to call it, brown adipose tissue). It was believed that this brown fat, which helps infants survive by protecting them against the cold, disappeared—or least shrank to the point of being meaningless—when we become adults. And second, because brown fat is a very unique type of fat. (See box on page 147: What Makes Brown Fat Tick?) Unlike white fat (white apidose tissue)—which makes up the vast majority of the fat in our bodies and is used to store any excess calories we consume—brown fat actually *burns* calories to produce heat under the right conditions. In fact, when fully activated, brown fat generates three hundred times more heat than any other tissue in the body. Just two ounces of brown fat appear capable of burning several hundred calories per day—the equivalent of a thirty-minute bout of exercise.

Although the news that at least some adults have brown fat was exciting, it wasn't clear at first how valuable this information would be. After all, if only a sliver of the population had brown fat deposits, the discovery wasn't likely to have any widespread applications in terms of health and wellness. We're now finding evidence, however, that most, and perhaps all, adults have small pockets of brown fat. The first hints of this came in two other smaller studies published around the same time as Dr. Cypess's, suggesting that the actual percentage of adults with brown fat was much higher than what their numbers indicated. That's because the scans reviewed by Dr. Cypess and Dr. Kahn were all done at more or less room temperature. But brown fat, by its very nature, is only "turned on" in cooler temperatures.

In one of the studies, investigators in the Netherlands scanned twenty-four men after they'd spent two hours in a room cooled to 60.8° F (16°C) and found that all but one had detectable deposits of brown fat. In another study, Swedish researchers scanned five subjects after they'd spent two hours at temperatures ranging from 63°F to 66°F. During the scan itself, the subjects cooled their body temperature even further by repeatedly placing one foot in ice water for five minutes at a time, followed by five minutes out of the water. The investigators found not only that all the subjects had detectable brown fat deposits but that the added exposure to the cold ice water boosted their brown-fat activity fifteen-fold.

These results indicated that most people have brown fat and that this brown fat springs into activity during exposure to cold. But again, because most people aren't inclined to take frigid foot baths, it was unclear how useful these findings were.

Despite these apparent obstacles, Dr. Cypess persevered, inspired by his own findings and those of the other research groups. In searching for a convenient way to reliably activate brown fat, he struck on the idea of taking cooling vests—vests containing tubelike compartments that can be filled with cold water, which are often worn by surgeons and their surgical teams to keep from overheating during long procedures under the hot lights of the operating room—and using them on research subjects in order to activate their brown fat stores. After some trial and error (including initial experiments on himself), Dr. Cypess found that filling the vest with 57°F water was ideal for activating brown fat, being cool enough to turn on the fat's heat-generating process without being so cold that subjects would start to shiver.

Since then, repeated experiments have shown that within just five minutes of donning the vests, brown fat activity starts showing up in 95% of test subjects. These results, which Dr. Cypess published recently, have helped establish brown fat's potential as a bona fide weight-loss mechanism.

"As a physician, I have many patients whose weight keeps creeping back up to a certain point, no matter how hard they try to lose those unwanted pounds," says Dr. Cypess. "Brown fat may help to down-shift the body's set point." This set point is the level of body weight at which the brain automatically begins to slow down metabolic activity, making it more difficult to lose additional weight. "If brown fat can lower the point where your brain thinks your body weight should be, it could turn out to be an important mechanism for boosting daily energy expenditure and keeping weight loss off," adds Dr. Cypess.

Brown Fat Enhances Glucose Metabolism

The calorie-burning potential of brown fat is exciting in and of itself, particularly because losing weight is so important for people with type 2 diabetes. But brown fat may have other diabetes-fighting properties as well: People with lower glucose levels tend to have more brown fat than those with higher levels, indicating that it may play a more direct role in glucose control. One group of investigators, for example, recently found that a certain protein in brown fat appears to enhance the metabolism of white fat. When they studied a strain of experimental mice who were lacking this protein, the mice expended less energy, gained weight, and developed diabetes.

In another research project, conducted here at Joslin in Dr. Laurie Goodyear's section on Integrative Physiology and Metabolism, a team headed by Dr. Kristin Stanford transplanted a small amount of brown fat from one group of mice into the abdomens of another group. The results of the study were astonishing: After eight weeks, the mice given the transplants were not only leaner than a placebo group, but also processed blood glucose better and had reduced insulin resistance. In a subsequent experiment, mice with brown fat transplants who were put on a high-fat diet had less weight gain and better glucose control than a placebo group. Further testing showed that the mice in the transplant group had elevated levels of various proteins and other substances that are important for blood glucose control.

Equally intriguing is the possibility that we may be able to grow additional brown fat cells in our body. In another groundbreaking piece of research, a team of basic scientists at Joslin led by Dr. Yu-Hua Tseng identified the adult stem cells that turn into brown fat and developed a way to extract these progenitor cells from both white fat and muscle tissue and coax them to grow into brown fat cells. Drs. Tseng and Cypess have also joined forces to begin teasing out the molecular pathways that are involved in the growth of brown fat cells. Researchers are also studying beige fat, which differs slightly from brown fat in its physiology but burns calories almost as effectively as brown fat does.

All of this innovative brown and beige fat research being conducted at Joslin and elsewhere means that we're certain to be hearing more news about this fascinating tissue in the years ahead. In fact, I think there's a reasonable chance that some form of personalized brown fat therapy may emerge at some point in the future, at least for those able to afford it. In the meantime, though, we already know enough to suggest some very inexpensive ways for you to maximize the activity of your own brown fat. In the next section, I'll explain how to do this.

How to Increase Your Own Brown Fat Activity

Although some people have dismissed brown fat as a biological novelty, I believe its promise as an important tool for fighting type 2 diabetes and obesity is very real. If someone is able to burn an extra two or three hundred calories per day, that's enough to shed a pound of body fat in just a couple of weeks. As Americans get older, we typically add ten pounds of weight per decade. The calorie-burning boost from brown fat could be enough to reverse this weight gain and help older individuals maintain the body weight they had as young adults. By revving up metabolic activity, brown fat could also help combat the metabolic slowdown that occurs when people start dieting—the set point phenomenon described previously, which is one of the most difficult obstacles to losing weight.

Activating your brown fat is probably not going to bring someone from an obese state to a healthy body weight on its own, but if brown fat activation is combined with exercise and diet, it could make a major difference in terms of helping the one fourth of the U.S. population who are significantly overweight drop down to a normal, healthy weight.

One thing that's clear from studies done so far, though, is that you have to find a way to trigger activity in your brown fat cells in order to experience their calorie-burning effect. On the other hand, as Dr. Cypess has shown in his cool-vest experiments, under the right conditions, activation of your brown fat can occur very quickly. Here are some suggested ways to stimulate your own brown fat cells to begin burning calories. As always, I want to stress that everyone's physiology is slightly different and that some of these approaches may work better for you than others.

EXPOSE YOUR SKIN TO COOLER TEMPERATURES

The most proven way to activate brown fat is to expose your skin to relatively cool temperatures. Colder temperatures send a signal to your brain, which then acts to stimulate brown fat activity in two ways: by acting on your vascular system directly to increase blood flow to your brown fat stores and by sending nerve impulses to brown fat cells that stimulate an additional boost in cellular activity.

How cool do you have to be? In addition to their studies with vests containing 57°F water, Drs. Kahn and Cypess have also found that sitting in a 59°F room for two hours wearing summer clothing will stimulate brown fat to burn an extra 100 to 250 calories, depending on the individual. A Japanese research team put subjects in an even milder setting of 66°F, and found that more than half of subjects under age thirty-eight showed signs of brown fat activation. (For the over-thirty-eight group the results were less impressive, with fewer than 10% showing any brown fat effect.) In another study conducted by a group of Canadian researchers, subjects wearing a suit containing tubes filled with 64°F water burned about 250 extra calories over three hours, most of which appeared to be the result of increased brown fat activity.

WHAT TO DO

These experiments indicate that lowering the thermostat of your residence to the mid-60s or below may be enough to stimulate at least some brown fat activity. You can also activate your brown fat by dressing more lightly in cool weather. For people willing to expose themselves to even cooler temperatures, a number of cooling vests are available (see box on page 144: Cooling Vests for Brown Fat Activation). In fact, our Joslin group is working on their own version right now. Research is also now underway to investigate whether exposing just one part of the body to cooler temperatures (by wearing a cooling band around your arm or leg, for example) might be enough to stimulate brown fat activity.

Activity Tip: You can boost the amount of calories you burn during exercise by stimulating your brown fat stores during your workout. Make a point of exercising in relatively cool temperatures—62°F to 64°F or lower. Making sure your skin is exposed while you're exercising may be even more beneficial because the evaporation of sweat as you exercise adds to the cooling effect. What you *don't* want to do is try to increase how much you perspire by turning up the heat when you're exercising because this hotter environment will actually shut down brown fat activity.

FOODS THAT MAY ACTIVATE YOUR BROWN FAT

Although there's no firm evidence that any specific foods or nutrients can activate brown fat, it's interesting to note that radiologists—who want to *decrease* brown fat activity when doing scans of cancer patients because the heat generated by activated brown fat makes it harder to see tumor-related activity—routinely recommend that patients eat a high-fat, low-carbohydrate diet before such scans, on the grounds that this *reduces* brown fat activation. This suggests, of course, that eating a low-fat, high-carbohydrate diet (like the RAD eating plan recommended in Strategy Chapter 1) will *boost* brown fat activity.

In addition, animal studies have found that the herb bitter melon appears to increase activity of brown fat and that ursolic acid—a substance that occurs in high concentrations in apple peels—increases brown fat *and* muscle mass, while at the same time reducing obesity and improving glucose tolerance. Other foods containing ursolic acid include cranberries, blueberries, plums, and prunes, as well as the herbs oregano, thyme, lavender, holy basil, bilberry, devil's claw, peppermint leaves, periwinkle, and hawthorn. Ursolic acid is also available in supplement form.

Cooling Vests for Brown Fat Activation

Here is a sampling of the various cooling vests on the market. The following products generally cost in the range of $200 or less.

- *RPCM Cool Vest for Therapy.* Cooling method: Phase-change technology (inserts that absorb body heat). Glacier Tek. (800) 482-0533; coolvest.com

- *Personal Microclimate Body Cooling Vest.* Cooling method: Circulating chilled liquid. Veskimo. (877) 698-3754. veskimo.com

- *Stacool Under Vest.* Cooling method: Reusable cold pack inserts. Stacool Industries. (866) 782-2665. stacoolvest.com

- *CoolVest Phase Change Cooling Vest.* Cooling method: Phase-change technology. Miller Therapeutic Cooling Products. (800) 728-1998. coolingtherapy.com

- *Aqua Vest Active.* Cooling method: Circulating ice water plus evaporative cooling. Miller Therapeutic Cooling Products. (800) 728-1998. coolingtherapy.com

- *Kool Max Cooling Vests.* Cooling method: Reusable cold pack inserts. Polar Products. (800) 763-8423. polarproducts.com

- *Arctic Heat Body Cooling Vest.* Cooling method: Cold gel pockets. Arctic Heat USA. arcticheatusa.com

EXERCISE

Although the benefits of exercise for your cardiovascular health, glucose control, and weight management are well known, researchers are now discovering that working out may have a positive effect on brown fat activity as well: Studies have found that irisin, a newly identified hormone that is produced during exercise, actually works to convert white fat into a variation of brown fat known as beige fat (see next page).

These findings show that both brown and beige fat can burn calories and, even more exciting, that the two types of fat are activated in different ways—with cool temperatures inducing brown fat to become active and exercise transforming white fat into beige fat. This suggests that there are actually multiple ways to increase your calorie-burning fats and reduce the amount of unhealthy, calorie-storing white fat in your body.

Where Is Brown Fat Stored?

Although the exact location of brown fat deposits in adults varies somewhat from individual to individual, PET-CT scans show that these deposits are typically located in the sides of the neck—sometimes running down into the shoulders and upper arms—and in the region just above the collarbone. Other common locations include the upper back between the shoulder blades and along the sides of the upper spine. Brown fat may also be found around the large blood vessels of the chest and, to a lesser extent, around the kidneys.

The actual amount of brown fat in these deposits generally adds up to a couple of ounces at most. Because they are so small and lie deep under the skin, they don't appear as bulges, like love handles, and don't have anything to do with what's commonly thought of as being "fat." Experimental data suggest that brown fat is more prevalent in younger adults and people who are lean, but it's not clear whether individuals who are older or overweight actually have less brown fat or simply have brown fat stores that are relatively dormant. To date, our ability to pinpoint people's brown fat locations has been hampered by the fact that PET and CT scans expose people to relatively high levels of radiation, limiting how often they can be used on any one person. Joslin researcher Aaron Cypess is now working with the famous Draper Lab at the Massachusetts Institute of Technology to develop a handheld infrared scanner that can detect active brown fat instantly through the heat it generates, without exposing subjects to any radiation whatsoever. Eventually, it may be possible to wear a personal infrared monitor while you're exercising— allowing you to check your own brown fat activity as you work out!

Is "Beige" the New Brown?

As we learn more about brown fat, a new category known as "beige" fat is also coming into focus. The term brings some confusion with it, however, because it is currently used interchangeably by various researchers in reference to what are really two different types of fat deposits. Some researchers use this term to describe tissue where small deposits of brown fat are interspersed inside white fat stores, creating a mixture of brown and white fat that is lighter in color than larger, concentrated deposits of brown fat. Researchers have also identified what appears to be a truly unique type of beige fat cell that is halfway between brown and white fat. The data seem to suggest this type of beige fat is more like brown fat from a genetic perspective and may in fact be an early stage form of brown fat. Most important, it has much the same calorie-burning effect that brown fat does.

The existence of this intermediate form of brown fat as well as the existence of small brown fat deposits inside larger white fat stores both suggest that beige fat may either have started out as white fat cells that have somehow been transformed into beige cells or derive from adult stem cells located in the white fat. Our scientists find both hypotheses exciting because they raise the possibility that we may one day be able to use our white fat stores as a resource for growing more brown fat cells.

Inside Joslin: The Search for a Brown Fat Drug

Given brown fat's powerful ability to burn calories and white fat, one tantalizing thought is that it might be possible to develop a medication that stimulates brown fat activity or perhaps even grows new brown fat cells. At last count, at least four companies were looking at a number of different approaches, but none have panned out yet.

Other studies here at Joslin have yielded more promising results, however. In 2008, a year before the wave of studies reporting the discovery of brown fat in adult humans, Dr. Tseng and her colleagues published a study showing that BMP-7, a drug administered after spinal fracture surgery to promote bone growth, promoted the growth of brown fat from progenitor cells when it was injected into mice. She and Dr. Cypess are now investigating whether brown fat stores are increased in people receiving BMP-7 treatment following spinal surgery. Dr. Tseng's lab has also shown that exposing white fat cells from mice to the diabetes drug rosiglitazone (Avandia) increases the rate at which progenitor cells in the fat are converted into brown fat—suggesting that this medication may have a future as a brown fat booster as well.

What Makes Brown Fat Tick?

As you might expect from its behavior, the biological makeup of brown fat is different from white fat in a number of ways. Some of these differences account for its color, which actually ranges from dark red to tan. Brown fat cells contain an unusually high number of mitochondria—tiny chemical factories whose functions include converting oxygen and nutrients such as glucose and fatty acids into either energy (in most cells) or heat (in brown fat cells). We discussed in Strategy Chapter 3 how impairments in mitochondrial function—a decrease in the ability of these tiny cellular energy factories to oxidize glucose, fatty acids, and other fuels—appear to be one of the contributing factors to insulin resistance in the muscles. In brown fat, on the other hand, mitochondria contribute not only to its calorie-burning properties but also its appearance: Mitochondria are rich in iron, which gives them a brown coloring. Brown fat tissue also contains many more of the tiny blood vessels known as capillaries than white fat does. These blood vessels add a reddish hue to brown fat cells. A final reason for brown fat's color is that each cell contains a smaller volume of lipids—the actual "fat" in fat cells, which is yellowish in color—than white fat does.

Brown fat is also rich in nerves, which transmit signals from the brain that trigger brown fat's heat-generating activity. Researchers at Joslin and other labs are now hard at work uncovering the mechanisms that enable this activity to occur. One important player is a protein called UCP-1, which brown fat is exceptionally high in. As noted previously, mitochondria usually convert oxygen and nutrients into cell-powering energy, in the form of a molecule called ATP (adenosine triphosphate). UCP-1 interferes with the ATP manufacturing process, however, causing the mitochondria in brown fat to produce heat instead.

As a result of all these features, brown fat is capable of producing heat at a much, much higher rate than other tissues, making it ideally designed to warm the body. This is why it accounts for about 5% of total weight in newborn babies, who are especially vulnerable to cold. And because the heat it produces uses up the fatty acids inside its cells, which are then replenished by drawing on white fat stores—a process recently confirmed by a group of Canadian researchers—it's perfectly designed to help adults reduce their body fat and maintain a healthy weight as well.

In the near future, I predict there will be multiple ways to activate and increase your brown fat stores, including working out in cool temperature rooms while monitoring your brown fat activity in real time and wearing a temperature-regulated vest or cooling patches or bands designed to maintain the activation of brown fat in warm weather or during exercise. It's also possible that there will be pharmaceutical stimulants that will not only activate your existing brown fat but also increase the amount of brown fat in your body. Last, there may one day be a way to convert unhealthy excess white fat to health-promoting brown fat—the holy grail of brown fat researchers.

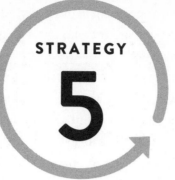

TURN YOUR BODY INTO AN INFLAMMATION-FIGHTING MACHINE

In recent years, scientists have come to understand that chronic, low-grade inflammation, caused by excessive body fat as well as other sources of infection or tissue damage in the body—with symptoms ranging from the bleeding gums of periodontal disease to the digestive distress of irritable bowel syndrome to the dry, flaky skin of psoriasis—is a significant contributor to insulin resistance. By following the advice in this chapter and treating and eliminating these sources of chronic inflammation, you will help boost your insulin sensitivity, protect the insulin-producing cells in your pancreas from damage, and improve your ability to metabolize glucose.

Every year, I give talks to various groups about the importance of good dental hygiene in preventing or managing diabetes and prediabetes. Are you surprised to hear that your body's ability to metabolize glucose can be affected by how well or poorly you floss and brush your teeth and gums? In fact, studies have found that preventing gum disease from taking hold in your mouth may make the management of your prediabetes or type 2 diabetes easier. The connection between the two represents one more facet in our growing understanding of how inflammation impacts glucose metabolism—a discovery that has taken nearly 150 years to play out.

To explain what I mean, let me back up for a moment. Although we think of scientific discovery as an inevitable march forward toward greater knowledge, not too infrequently, a significant finding is made and then forgotten, waiting for future investigators to rediscover it. Well over a century ago, physicians began reporting that when they gave potent doses of sodium salicylate—a salt close in chemical form to aspirin that contains similar anti-inflammatory properties—to patients with adult onset diabetes, their symptoms lessened considerably. Early in the twentieth century, however, that insight vanished into the medical archives. It was resurrected briefly in the late 1950s, when another group of physicians noticed that if they treated a diabetic patient with high-dose aspirin to relieve arthritis symptoms brought on by rheumatic fever, the patient no longer required daily insulin shots. They proceeded to give a small group of diabetic patients a high-dose aspirin for two weeks and found their fasting blood glucose levels dropped from 192 mg/dL to 92 mg/dL, on average. Because no one understood the mechanism underlying this effect and because such a high dose of aspirin was required, however, the discovery again fell by the wayside.

The idea that chronic, low-grade inflammation is a major contributor to insulin resistance and type 2 diabetes risk finally surfaced as a serious theory in the 1990s. Over the past twenty years, Joslin investigators, led by Dr. Steven Shoelson and Dr. Allison Goldfine, have helped establish the inflammation-insulin resistance connection as an important new frontier in diabetes research. In one key finding, Dr. Shoelson's lab discovered that the molecule NF-κB, an important immune-system regulator found in fat and liver tissue, is activated by obesity and a high-fat diet and is a contributor to insulin resistance. Then, in a 2001 study, they showed that aspirin can improve insulin sensitivity in genetically obese mice by blocking the protein IKK-β pathway, which plays an important role in the signaling cascade that produces NF-κB. During this time, Dr. Shoelsen's lab also rediscovered the literature on sodium salicylate and determined that one of its main mechanisms of action was also to inhibit the activity of NF-κB. (My own lab is currently studying the role of NF-κB and inflammation as part of the molecular process involved in diabetic eye disease.)

High-dose aspirin has too many dangerous side effects to be an effective treatment for diabetes and prediabetes. Dr. Shoelson and Dr. Goldfine are now, however, breaking new ground with clinical trials testing the antidiabetes effects of another safer alternative to aspirin called salsalate, a type of salicylate that is a close relative of the centuries-old remedy sodium salicylate. (See box on page 160: Inside Joslin: Is Salsalate the New/Old Diabetes Wonder Drug?)

Today it's becoming widely accepted that when chronic, low-grade inflammation develops, it plays an important contributing role in both insulin resistance and the development of type 2 diabetes. Therefore, decreasing this inflammation is a key to boosting your insulin sensitivity. It's important to note, too, that low-grade inflammation has been shown to contribute to other important diseases as well, including atherosclerosis, or hardening of the arteries.

What Causes Chronic, Low-Grade Inflammation and Six Ways to Prevent It

I n the strategy chapter on weight loss, I discuss how the inflammatory effects of excess body fat contribute to insulin resistance—and specifically, how inflammatory molecules called cytokines interfere with the complex signaling process that insulin uses to metabolize glucose molecules. Being overweight is just one potential source of inflammation, however. Many other medical conditions, including gum infections, cardiovascular disease, and autoimmune disorders like psoriasis, inflammatory bowel disease, or celiac disease can also contribute to chronic, low-grade inflammation throughout your body, leading your immune system to pump out pro-inflammatory molecules that can interfere with the insulin-signaling process just as obesity-related inflammation does.

Although this chronic, low-grade inflammation doesn't cause the obvious redness, pain, and swelling that we associate with acute inflammation, it can significantly reduce your body's insulin sensitivity. The treatment of chronic inflammation is now emerging as an important new frontier in the fight to prevent and reverse diabetes, prediabetes, and many other chronic diseases. I've already mentioned that losing weight and getting sufficient sleep will help keep inflammation at bay. Here are some other anti-inflammatory measures you can take that will help enhance your body's ability to metabolize blood glucose and improve your overall health.

1. GET YOUR C-REACTIVE PROTEIN (CRP) LEVELS CHECKED.

C-reactive protein, commonly abbreviated as CRP, is a blood protein that rises sharply and quickly in response to infection and in the presence of inflammatory cytokines such as TNF-α, IL-6, and IL-1. This property makes it an excellent marker for inflammation. When there is unresolved infection or activation of immune reactions in the body, CRP can become persistently elevated to a small degree, signaling that there is a chronic source of inflammation in the body.

An inexpensive and highly accurate blood test for CRP has been available for some time and has come into wide use as a tool for gauging heart attack risk—because, as noted previously, cardiovascular disease and particularly atherosclerosis are associated with chronic inflammation of the blood vessels. Recent

How to Interpret Your CRP Test Results

- Less than 1 milligram per liter (mg/L) of CRP in the blood is considered normal, indicating a low risk for insulin resistance and heart attack.

- A CRP level of 1 to 3 mg/L has been associated with an elevated risk of insulin resistance in some studies, as well as a moderate risk of heart attack.

- A CRP level above 3 mg/L is associated with high risk of insulin resistance and heart attack.

- A CRP level over 10 mg/L typically indicates an active infection or inflammatory disease, which is a separate issue from low-grade, chronic inflammation. You'll need to follow up by consulting with your doctor on why you might have such high CRP levels. A follow-up CRP test is recommended once symptoms subside.

studies have shown that blood levels of C-reactive protein also corre-late closely with insulin resistance and type 2 diabetes risk. Elevation of CRP can be an important warning sign of problems with your glucose metabolism, even in the absence of obesity. For this reason, I recom-mend having regular CRP readings taken—every four to six months, if possible—to follow the effects of the interventions outlined in this book, including diet, exercise, or other treatments to lower inflammation. In fact, your CRP levels will provide you with a more sensitive indication of your inflammatory status and related improvements in glucose metabo-lism than actual weight loss will.

A CRP blood test is simple to do, requiring a very small blood draw, and typically costs less than $20 when ordered through your doctor from a lab under insurance coverage. These days, it is often included in the battery of blood tests given as part of an annual physical exam. I highly recommend that you ask your primary care physician to test your CRP levels on a regular basis if you're not getting this done already.

WHAT TO DO. If your CRP levels are elevated or are higher than they were previously, you should discuss your results with your doctor. Researchers have found that CRP levels can be lowered through many of the strategies outlined in this book, including losing weight, getting regular aerobic exercise, eating a diet low in fat and high in fiber, treating minor but persistent infections, and improving sleep duration or patterns. At the same time, you should also pay close attention to the other inflammation-fighting tips in this chapter.

2. DON'T SMOKE.

Believe it or not, some 20% of the U.S. population still smokes. A num-ber of studies have clearly shown that smoking cigarettes increases risk of developing type 2 diabetes. The Nurses' Health Study, which followed 114,000 women for two decades, found that, after accounting for all other risk factors, those who smoked were 1.4 times more likely to develop type 2 diabetes than nonsmokers. Large-scale studies in Korea, Japan, and Britain have found a similar link, with diabetes risk increasing in proportion to the number of cigarettes smoked daily. Smoking has also been shown to induce insulin resistance in both type 2 diabetics and healthy individuals, and studies in the United Kingdom and Sweden have found that smokers have higher hemoglobin A1C levels than non-smokers. Smokers with type 2 diabetes are also at greater risk for certain diabetic complications than diabetic patients who don't smoke, including kidney disease and cardiovascular disease.

Smoking appears to disrupt glucose metabolism in a number of ways; it raises levels of fatty acids in the bloodstream—which promotes insulin resistance in the skeletal muscles—and also increases oxidative stress and blood levels of the stress hormone cortisol, both of which can interfere with insulin signaling. Nicotine itself seems to be a factor as well because increased insulin resistance has been noted in people who chew nicotine gum. Cigarette smoking also leads to chronic, systemic inflammation: Studies have linked smoking to elevated CRP levels as well as increased blood levels of interleukin-6—a pro-inflammatory cytokine, which, as previously noted, is known to interfere with insulin signaling—and other pro-inflammatory molecules. To cite one startling indication of just how powerful the inflammatory effects of smoking are, researchers have found that CRP levels remain elevated in former cigarette smokers *for ten to twenty years* after they've quit smoking! Lastly, in people with diabetes, smoking can dramatically increase their risk of heart and peripheral disease much more than it does in nondiabetic people because smoking actually *multiplies* the threat of other risk factors rather than simply adding to them.

WHAT TO DO. If you are experiencing problems with blood glucose control, you should avoid smoking completely. If you are a habitual smoker, then you should make a concerted effort to quit. Rather than try to quit on your own, I recommend that you consult with a clinician who specializes in helping smokers quit or join a formal smoking cessation program. A combination of individual, group, or telephone counseling, particularly counseling that involves problem solving, skills training, and social support, together with medication, has been shown to be especially effective. First-line medications that are proven to result in long-term abstinence include nicotine formulations—nicotine gum, patches, lozenges, inhalers, and nasal spray—and the medications Vernicline and Bupropion SR.

For more information on how to quit, visit the website smokefree .gov. You can also talk to a trained counselor from the National Cancer Institute from 8 a.m. to 8 p.m. Eastern Time, Monday through Friday, by calling 877-44U-QUIT (877-448-7848), or speak with a trained smoking-cessation coach in your home state by calling 800-QUIT-NOW (800-784-8669).

3. PREVENT GUM DISEASE THROUGH GOOD DENTAL HYGIENE—AND IF YOU DO DEVELOP GUM DISEASE, SEEK PROMPT TREATMENT FOR IT.

The gums, with their continual exposure to food and liquid, are one of the most common sources of chronic inflammation. It is estimated that about one out of three Americans has some evidence of periodontal (gum) disease and that one third of this group has full-blown gum infections, in which toxic, anaerobic (nonoxygen-using) bacteria invades the pockets between the gum and the teeth. Infections of the gum pockets are particularly worrisome for people at risk of type 2 diabetes because the immune system often can't eliminate this type of infection on its own. As a result, the infection festers, the immune system remains permanently activated, and chronic inflammation sets in. Worse still, both the bacteria from gum disease and the cytokines the immune system secretes to fight them—including TNF-α and IL-6, both of which have been shown to interfere with the action of insulin—can readily pass from the gum tissue into the bloodstream, spreading these pro-inflammatory molecules throughout the body. In addition, gum disease (periodontal disease) is a major cause for losing teeth,

> ### Warning Signs of Gum Disease
>
> - Bleeding while brushing (look for the telltale pink hue on your toothbrush)
> - Red, swollen, or tender gums
> - A receding gum line
> - Loose teeth
> - Chronic bad breath
> - A change in your bite pattern or the fit of your dentures

which in turn makes people choose a diet containing food with lighter texture and less fiber. This type of food tends to be high in calories and fat content—which, as I discuss elsewhere in this book, promotes obesity, inflammation, and diabetes.

A number of studies have linked gum disease to increased risk of insulin resistance and type 2 diabetes. In one 2008 study conducted at Columbia University, researchers reviewed twenty years' worth of data on a sample of more than nine thousand people, none of whom had diabetes at the start of the study. They found that, after accounting for factors such as smoking, diet, and body weight, those with periodontal infections were almost twice as likely to develop type 2 diabetes over the ensuing twenty years.

On the other hand, treatment of gum disease may also reduce systemic inflammation and improve blood glucose control. In a 2005 study, patients with well-controlled type 2 diabetes who underwent periodontal treatment for gum disease recorded a statistically significant improvement in their glucose control three months later, as measured by their hemoglobin A1C levels, while a matched control group that had no periodontal treatment for their gum health showed no improvement. Another study of individuals with type 2 diabetes and periodontal disease, published in 2001, found that periodontal treatment led to reductions in blood levels of the pro-inflammatory cytokine TNF-α *and* hemoglobin A1C levels. It also found that the amount of improvement in blood glucose control correlated closely with the degree of TNF-α reduction across the study population.

It should be noted that not all such studies have shown that improving gum disease will improve glucose control. It is likely, however, that significant improvement of severe gum disease will make maintenance of diabetes care easier. In addition, it is clear that diabetes itself increases the risk for periodontal disease and loss of teeth. Again, this loss of teeth can affect nutrition by decreasing the intake of high-fiber food. Clearly, changes in diet will alter bacteria flora not only in the mouth but also in the gut and affect total body health statistics.

WHAT TO DO. To keep your gums healthy, brush at least twice a day with a fluoride toothpaste, including just before going to bed; floss after each meal; and use a fluoride, antiplaque, or antiseptic mouthwash. For those who are at risk for periodontal disease, the use of interdental soft picks is also recommended. An electric toothbrush cleans more effectively than a manual one, and brushing along the gum line with diluted hydrogen peroxide can also help destroy any bacteria that are present. Avoid smoking cigarettes, which can increase your risk of gum disease by up to six times, and eat a nutritious diet with minimal intake of foods containing sugar. Finally, be sure to see your dentist regularly for an exam and cleaning.

If your gums show signs of inflammation, consult with your dentist to see whether you require treatment from a periodontist. This treatment typically involves a professional cleaning of the teeth and gums, debriding (scraping away) the infected gum tissue, and administering both topical antimicrobial agents and systemic antibiotics.

4. AVOID BREATHING SMOKE, SMOG, AND CAR EXHAUST.

Recently, new evidence has emerged linking the inflammation caused by breathing in particles found in smog and car exhaust with increased risk of developing insulin resistance and type 2 diabetes. Particulates with a size between 1 and 2.5 micrometers (a unit, also known as a micron, that is one-thousandth of a millimeter) pose particular risk because they're small enough to penetrate deep into the lungs and other organs. These types of particulates, classified as PM2.5, are the main component of haze, smoke, and car exhaust. In one recently published study, on which Joslin's Dr. Allison Goldfine was a co-investigator, researchers looked at every county in the U.S., comparing the data on average PM2.5 levels to the rates of diabetes. After controlling for other diabetes risk factors, they found that counties with the highest PM2.5 levels, although still being within the EPA acceptable exposure limits, had more than 20% higher rates of type 2 diabetes than counties with the lowest PM2.5 levels.

This finding is reinforced by other research, including an animal study showing that exposure to higher levels of air pollution leads to increased fat accumulation and inflammation and increased insulin resistance in mice who are fed a normal diet, as well as studies showing increased blood markers for inflammation among people with type 2 diabetes who are exposed to higher levels of PM2.5. Exposure to PM2.5 has also been linked to increased risk of vascular inflammation and atherosclerosis (hardening of the arteries).

WHAT TO DO. You can check the air quality in your home county, including the amount of particulate matter, by visiting the American Lung Association's "State of the Air" website at stateoftheair.org. Short of moving to an area with lower PM2.5 levels, you can wear an N95 respiratory mask while outdoors. These are masks that have been certified to remove at least 95% of the particulate matter from the air you breathe. It's important to use only a mask with a NIOSH (National Institute of Occupational Safety and Health) N95 certification (the dust masks you can buy in a hardware store look similar, but are much less effective). A list of certified N95 masks can be found by going to the Centers for Disease Control Prevention website at cdc.gov and typing "N95" into the site's search engine.

To remove air particulates from your indoor spaces (where adults spend 90% of their time) use either a HEPA (high-energy particulate air) filter—the best ones remove nearly 100% of particles down to a size as small as 0.3 microns—or an electrostatic air filter that draws air particles through a chamber where they are given an electric charge, then traps them against plates with an opposite charge. You should also avoid exercising outdoors in smoggy or sooty environments because studies suggest that this leads to higher accumulations of soot in the lungs.

5. EAT FOODS THAT FIGHT INFLAMMATION.

The Rural Asian Diet contains many foods that have been found to have anti-inflammatory benefits. Following are a number of examples of these foods—all of which are part of the RAD eating plan outlined in Strategy Chapter 1. Because everyone's body chemistry is slightly different, as you bring these foods into your daily diet, keep track of how specific foods affect any inflammatory conditions you may have.

WHAT TO DO. Incorporate as many of these foods as possible into your daily menu. As you eat a meal rich in any one of these food types, keep track of any inflammatory conditions you may have to see if they are reduced. If so, continue to emphasize that food in your meal planning.

- Fatty fish (e.g., salmon, tuna, sardines)

- Whole grains and whole-grain products

- Vegetables, especially colorful fruits and cruciferous vegetables (e.g., broccoli, Brussels sprouts, cauliflower)

- Mushrooms

- Fruits. These should be enjoyed in a variety of colors (e.g., raspberries, blueberries, cherries, grapefruit) because each color represents a different array of healing biochemicals.

- Nuts

- Legumes

- Soy and soy products

- Garlic

- Onions

- Heart healthy oil (e.g., olive oil, canola oil)

Signs of Other Chronic Inflammatory Conditions

- *Diarrhea, abdominal pain and cramping, and bloody stools.* These are all potential symptoms of Crohn's disease, a condition in which the intestine becomes inflamed, as well as colitis, marked by inflammation of the colon.

- *Frequent need to urinate, pain or burning while urinating, smelly or cloudy urine, or lower abdominal pain.* These are all signs of a possible urinary tract infection, or UTI—an inflammation of the urethra or bladder, often caused by bacterial infection. People with elevated blood glucose are at higher risk for UTIs, in part because the urine then contains excess glucose as well, which can encourage bacterial infection.

- *Coughing, wheezing, chest tightness, shortness of breath.* These are all potential signs of asthma. A recent study by Mayo Clinic researchers found that the risk of developing type 2 diabetes was doubled among people with asthma compared to non-asthmatics.

- *Facial pain or pressure, persistent cough, nasal stuffiness or congestion, yellow or green nasal discharge.* These are signs of a chronic sinus inflammation.

• Tea. Green and black tea have been shown to have significant anti-inflammatory effects, with green tea being slightly superior—most likely because of its higher bioflavanoid content.

If you want to have a sweet treat, opt for dark chocolate, which has powerful anti-inflammatory properties thanks to its cocoa content. For the strongest effect, choose chocolate that is at least 65% cocoa. And if you drink alcohol, choose red wine, which some studies have shown has an anti-inflammatory action as well. Obviously, don't overindulge in either.

Inside Joslin: Is Salsalate the New (Old) Diabetes Wonder Drug?

One of the chief problems with popular anti-inflammatory medications like ibuprofen and naproxen, which inhibit both COX-1 and COX-2 enzymes, and selective COX-2 inhibitors such as Celebrex, which inhibit just COX-2, is that they affect other body functions besides inflammation. For example, COX enzymes also prevent the blood from clotting and the blood vessels from constricting and help maintain the stomach's protective lining of mucus. The suppression of these functions by such medications can give rise to problematic side effects when they're taken over time, including increased heart attack and stroke risk, high blood pressure, and stomach ulcers.

Aspirin (acetasylic acid), which has been shown to benefit blood glucose metabolism, suppresses COX enzymes in a different fashion. As a result, although it also suppresses production of protective mucus in the stomach lining, its effect on platelets is the opposite of the drugs mentioned previously: It actually impairs the ability of blood to clot, a fact that has made low-dose aspirin a daily must for people who want to prevent heart attack–causing clots, but that also leaves people at risk of uncontrolled bleeding when taken in high doses. It also suppresses production of mucus in the stomach lining as noted previously, leaving the stomach vulnerable to irritation from stomach acid.

Salicylates, although chemically related to aspirin, target inflammation by inhibiting NF-κB without affecting COX enzymes, meaning that they carry no risk of uncontrolled bleeding or stomach damage. Because salicylates have been shown to be effective at reducing blood glucose levels as well, there is now considerable interest in a generic salicylate drug called salsalate—a compound that is chemically very similar to the centuries-old

6. TAKE ANTI-INFLAMMATORY HERBAL SUPPLEMENTS.

Although anti-inflammatory medications such as NSAIDs (nonsteroidal anti-inflammatory drugs) and Cox-2 inhibitors can cause serious side effects, especially when used for an extended period of time, there are a number of herbs with anti-inflammatory properties that can help and are also very safe, having been used for centuries as spices for cooking.

remedy sodium salicylate, but better tolerated.

Joslin investigators Dr. Steven Shoelson and Dr. Allison Goldfine have been leading this effort. In a randomized clinical trial conducted at Joslin several years ago, 108 patients with type 2 diabetes were put on three different daily doses of salsalate or a placebo. All of those who took salsalate improved their triglyceride and blood sugar levels after three months, with those taking the highest dose—4 grams a day—reducing their hemoglobin A1C scores by an average of .5%. "We may have a new class of therapeutic agents to treat patients with type 2 diabetes," said Dr. Goldfine at the time. "When you have a new safe, effective, and inexpensive agent, that's pretty exciting."

In July 2013, the researchers published the Stage 2 results of the clinical trial, dubbed TINSAL-T2D (Targeting Inflammation Using Salsalate in Type 2 Diabetes). In this stage, they enrolled 286 participants whose type 2 diabetes was not adequately controlled by medication. After forty-eight weeks of treatment, the mean hemoglobin A1C level (a measurement of average blood glucose control over the prior twelve weeks) was 37% lower in the salsalate group compared to the placebo group. The decrease in fasting glucose concentration was also 15 mg/dL greater in the salsalate group than in the placebo group, and those in the salsalate group required fewer additional diabetes medications than patients in the placebo group. The salsalate group also reduced their triglycerides; showed a 27% increase in adiponectin, a protein secreted by fat cells that may potentially protect the cardiovascular system; and had reduced levels of several inflammatory markers, including circulating white blood cells and other immune system components called neutrophils and lymphocytes.

In addition to the ongoing diabetes trial, Dr. Goldfine is also currently leading a study to evaluate whether salsalate can improve coronary artery plaque volume in participants with established coronary artery disease. Clearly the "forgotten" salicylate remedies have come a long way.

TURMERIC/CURCUMIN. Curcumin is the active biological ingredient of turmeric root powder, an ingredient of curries and yellow mustard (brown and Dijon mustard don't contain turmeric). Curcumin has been found to have potent anti-inflammatory effects, and also stimulates production of the body's natural antioxidants. (For more on this latter benefit, see Strategy Chapter 8.) It inhibits the COX2 enzyme, a key pro-inflammatory substance that also is a target of many pharmaceutical anti-inflammatories, as well as eiconasoids, molecules that help mediate the body's inflammatory response.

Research indicates that taking curcumin supplements can reduce inflammation-related symptoms in people with rheumatoid arthritis

The Autoimmune Disorder–Diabetes Link

Could having an inflammatory autoimmune disease put you at greater risk for diabetes? In the case of at least one such disease, psoriasis, the answer appears to be yes. Like type 2 diabetes, psoriasis, which attacks the skin and other organs and affects 7.5 million Americans, is associated with chronic inflammation. An inflammatory pathway shared by both conditions, involving TH-1 cytokines, promotes both insulin resistance and the inflammatory cytokines known to drive psoriasis. When a recent study at the University of Pennsylvania compared 108,132 people with psoriasis to 430,716 matched patients without psoriasis, the researchers found that patients with mild psoriasis had an 11% increased risk of diabetes compared to those without psoriasis, whereas patients with severe psoriasis had a 46% greater risk. The investigators also found that patients with both psoriasis and diabetes were more likely to require diabetes medications than diabetics without the autoimmune disease.

Researchers are continuing to probe the biological links between diabetes and psoriasis as well as other autoimmune conditions. A recent analysis of population data by researchers at Brigham and Women's Hospital in Boston, for example, found that people with either psoriatic arthritis or rheumatoid arthritis had a 50% higher risk of developing diabetes than people without these conditions.

In the meantime, if you have an inflammatory autoimmune disease of any kind, be sure to get regular blood glucose screenings and work with a rheumatologist to control your inflammation-related symptoms.

even more effectively than a widely used NSAID. Animal studies have also found it to reduce inflammation from rheumatoid arthritis and slow the progression of osteoarthritis. There is also some evidence that it may inhibit the growth of amyloid plaque in the brain that has been associated with Alzheimer's disease.

Because curcumin is not readily absorbed by the body, you are best off trying curcumin supplements that have been modified to increase their absorption rates. High-absorption curcumin products include:

Curamin (Terry Naturally/EuroPharma), a supplement containing high-absorption curcumin combined with Boswellia, another herb with anti-inflammatory properties.

Biomor Curcumin (Healthy Source) and *Super Bio-Curcumin* (Life Extension), both of which have elements of turmeric root added back into them to increase absorption by the body.

Meriva (Thorne Research, Now Foods, Source Naturals), a supplement containing curcumin phytosome, a compound that combines curcumin with a human cell component to enhance its absorption rate.

Turmeric Curcumin TriForce (Tattva's Herbs), a product that combines two types of high-absorption curcumin extract with raw turmeric.

BOSWELLIA. Boswellia extract, derived from the resin of the boswellia serrata tree, reduces levels of pro-inflammatory leukotrienes and other molecules. It's been shown to help relieve colitis (inflammation of the digestive tract), as well as airway inflammation associated with asthma, and may reduce arthritis-related inflammation as well.

GINGER. Ginger, which is related to turmeric biologically, is often used to prevent nausea, but it also has potent anti-inflammatory properties. It works by inhibiting production of both COX1 and COX2 enzymes as well as other pro-inflammatory chemicals. Studies have shown that ginger extract supplements may be helpful in relieving arthritis-related knee pain. While consuming ginger tea or using fresh ginger in cooking may provide some mild anti-inflammatory benefits, studies of its inflammation-fighting properties have typically utilized powdered ginger root extract supplements, available from a wide variety of manufacturers both online and at pharmacies and health food stores.

ROSA CANINA. Research has shown that taking daily supplements of rosa canina extract for four weeks lowers CRP blood levels in both healthy individuals and those with osteoarthritis, and also provides moderate relief of arthritis symptoms. The extract, a type of rose hips obtained from a species of wild rose plant, appears to work by reducing the amount of neutrophils and other pro-inflammatory molecules in the peripheral tissues. It is also a rich source of vitamin C. Rosa canina extract is sold in capsule and powder form, including a patented version called *I-Flex* that is specifically formulated for arthritis relief. It is also available as a tea for milder anti-inflammatory benefits.

MULTI-HERB PRODUCTS. There are also a number of inflammation-reducing products that provide combinations of anti-inflammatory herbal extracts in capsule form. Here are two of the most popular:

- *Zyflamend* (New Chapter) containing rosemary, turmeric/curcumin, ginger, holy basil, green tea extract, Chinese knotweed, Chinese goldthread, barberry, oregano, Chinese skullcap, and several other anti-inflammatory compounds.

- *Inflammatone* (Designs for Health) containing turmeric/curcumin, boswellia, ginger, quercetin, rutin, rosemary, and Chinese knotweed.

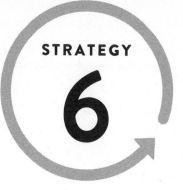

6

GET SEVEN TO EIGHT HOURS OF SLEEP EVERY NIGHT

There is growing evidence that lack of sufficient sleep—whether due to lifestyle or work schedule, difficulties falling or staying asleep, or the sleep-disordered breathing condition known as obstructive sleep apnea—can contribute to development of insulin resistance and may possibly cause damage to the pancreas as well, putting you at heightened risk for prediabetes and type 2 diabetes. By taking steps to ensure that you get a full, restful sleep each night, as outlined in this chapter, you can significantly improve your insulin sensitivity, help protect your beta cells, and lower your diabetes risk.

S everal years ago, my Joslin colleagues and I were privileged to get a visit from George M. Church, Ph.D., a professor of genetics at Harvard Medical School who is one of the world's leading molecular geneticists. Dr. Church helped develop DNA sequencing (the technology used to map out the genetic profiles of humans and other species) and was also one of the founders of the Human Genome Project. He had come to Joslin to learn more about our Gold Medalists— people who have lived with type 1 diabetes for more than fifty years after being diagnosed with their condition. Dr. Church was interested in understanding how this population's genetic makeup enabled them to survive so long with a condition that can potentially cause so many medical problems. During his visit, he explained that he had a similar interest in other long-lived groups and had spent a great deal of time studying centenarians (people who have lived to be 100 or older) and super-centenarians (those who are 110 or older).

As we spoke, the question arose: What might this group of century-old individuals have in common that allow them to live such long lives? "I'll tell you one thing," Dr. Church replied. "They all sleep very well at night."

In today's fast-paced world, a full night's sleep may seem like an impossible luxury. But there is a growing consensus in the medical world that lack of sleep can directly interfere with your body's ability to metabolize glucose. Over the past decade, diabetes researchers have been gathering a significant amount of evidence showing that insufficient or disrupted sleep increases your risk of developing prediabetes and type 2 diabetes, and also makes it harder to control your blood glucose levels if you do have one of these conditions.

In particular, lack of sleep appears to directly reduce insulin sensitivity in the body's peripheral tissues, thereby causing insulin resistance—which, as we've seen, is the primary underlying cause of prediabetes and type 2 diabetes. Chronic lack of sleep has also been linked to an increased risk of obesity—the main risk factor for type 2 diabetes—and increased activation of the body's stress response, which is another contributor to insulin resistance.

What the Studies Show

LABORATORY STUDIES

Although a number of studies had found that totally depriving subjects of sleep causes a rise in blood glucose levels, the first study attempting to simulate a more realistic "lack of sleep" scenario was done in 1999 at the University of Chicago and published in the *Lancet*. When eleven young, healthy men were allowed to sleep only four hours per night for six days, it took 40% longer for their blood glucose to drop to normal levels after

America's—and the World's—Growing Sleep Deficit

Over the past few decades, the amount of sleep that the average American gets each night has declined sharply. A 2011 analysis by the Centers for Disease Control and Prevention found that three out of ten Americans surveyed sleep less than seven hours a night on average. A similar report found that among middle-aged American adults, more than 30% indicated they were getting less than six hours per night! In addition, between 50 and 70 million people in the U.S. have chronic sleep disorders. Other surveys have found that Americans get one and a half to two hours less sleep per night now than they did forty years ago. During this same period, rates of type 2 diabetes and obesity have skyrocketed.

The problem of sleep deprivation isn't limited to the United States.

A number of studies have found dramatic levels of sleep deprivation in Westernized Asian cities—particularly Hong Kong and urban areas of Japan, Singapore, and China. Interestingly, before China liberalized its socialist economy, people tended to sleep well. Since the country introduced free-market principles, everyone has been working harder and sleeping less as a result. The fact that the three-thousand-mile-wide nation has just one time zone for everyone hasn't helped sleeping patterns either: It means all Chinese people must synchronize their lives even though the sun is rising three hours earlier in eastern China than it is in the western region of the country—causing some to wake consistently in darkness and go to sleep while it's still light.

eating a high-carbohydrate meal, and their ability to respond to insulin dropped by 30%, to a level comparable to that of much older individuals with diagnosed insulin resistance. They also showed increased activity of their sympathetic nervous system—the body's "fight or flight" response, which inhibits the release of insulin—and higher nighttime levels of the stress hormone cortisol, which actively counteracts the effects of insulin. These effects were reversed once the subjects were allowed to recover by sleeping twelve hours per night for a week.

Another important University of Chicago study, published in 2009 in the *Journal of Clinical Endocrinology and Metabolism,* took an even more realistic approach, recruiting eleven middle-aged individuals who didn't have diabetes but who were overweight and did little exercise. The subjects, who normally slept eight hours a night on average, were restricted to 5.5 hours of sleep per night for two weeks—equivalent to the amount of sleep many chronically sleep-deprived Americans usually get. By the end of the two-week period, the subjects' glucose tolerance (as measured by an oral glucose tolerance test) had declined significantly and so had their insulin sensitivity.

An even more recent study at Leiden University Medical Center in the Netherlands, published in 2010, found that a single night of sleeping only four hours was enough to reduce insulin sensitivity by 25%.

Especially convincing was a recent University of Chicago study, which put seven young, lean adults through four nights of just 4.5 hours of sleep per night, then measured insulin sensitivity in their fat cells directly and found these cells had become 30% less sensitive to the effects of insulin than at the start of the study—equivalent to the insulin sensitivity of people with full-blown diabetes.

POPULATION-BASED STUDIES

A number of population-based studies have also found a strong association between insufficient sleep and risk of prediabetes and type 2 diabetes.

An analysis of a cross-section of nearly 1,500 men and women in their fifties and older, taken from the Sleep Heart Health Study (SHHS), found that people who slept six hours or less per night had higher rates of diabetes and glucose intolerance than those who got between seven and eight hours of sleep nightly.

Similarly, the Massachusetts Male Aging Study, which followed 1,700 men ages forty to seventy for a decade and a half, found that those who slept six hours or less each night were twice as likely to develop diabetes as those who slept seven hours or more.

A more recent meta-analysis, published in 2010 by researchers at the University of Warwick in the United Kingdom, looked at data gathered on more than 107,000 subjects in ten previously conducted studies. It found that those who slept less than five or six hours on average (depending on the study) were 28% more likely to develop diabetes than those who slept six to eight hours per night.

How Lack of Sleep Affects Glucose Metabolism

All of this research naturally raises the question: What is it about getting too little sleep that makes someone's body less sensitive to insulin and less able to metabolize the glucose in his or her bloodstream? At this point, the answers to this question are somewhat speculative—but the prevailing thinking is that lack of sleep contributes to insulin resistance and glucose intolerance in a number of different ways. Indeed, the relationship between sleep and diabetes helps to reveal just how complex the human body's glucose metabolism process is and how many different factors can potentially contribute to the development of pre-diabetes and diabetes.

- One key mechanism that may contribute to insulin resistance in sleep-deprived individuals is an *increase in sympathetic nervous activity,* which has been shown to occur with lack of sleep. This increased activity boosts insulin resistance directly, through its neurologic effect on peripheral tissue, and also inhibits the body's release of insulin. In addition, there is growing evidence that sympathetic nervous activity impairs insulin sensitivity indirectly by triggering the release of pro-inflammatory cytokines—immune system components that can interfere with the insulin-signaling process, further contributing to insulin resistance. In fact, studies have shown that getting sufficient sleep exerts a neurologic effect that reduces overall inflammatory activity in the body, which, as we've seen, is now considered to be a major contributor to prediabetes and type 2 diabetes.

- Sleep deprivation also increases the body's production of the hormone cortisol, which counters the effects of insulin and increases insulin resistance by blocking the transport of glucose into the cells. At the same time, cortisol triggers the release of additional glucose from the liver, causing blood glucose levels to rise. (I'll discuss cortisol's detrimental effect on glucose metabolism at greater length in the next chapter.)

- Lack of sleep has also been linked to *increased levels of growth hormone,* which also contributes to insulin resistance by inhibiting insulin's ability to transport glucose into the peripheral tissues.

- The University of Chicago study mentioned previously, in which researchers detected reduced insulin sensitivity in the fat cells of the study's subjects, also identified a metabolic mechanism that may be partially to blame for the loss of insulin sensitivity. After losing sleep, the subjects all showed *impairment of a crucial step in the phosphatidylinositol 3-kinase (PI3K) pathway*—a complicated name for a very important chemical pathway that is vital to certain functions of insulin in the body. Two insulin functions disrupted by this change are the secretion of leptin, an appetite-suppressing hormone, and the metabolism of fatty acids. As a result, lack of sleep leaves the body with *lower levels of leptin*—making overeating more likely—and *higher levels of free fatty acids (FFAs),* which have been linked to insulin resistance in muscle tissue, as you'll recall from my discussion in Strategy Chapter 2 on how being overweight and eating a high-fat diet can combine to raise FFAs and lower insulin sensitivity.

- The increase in sympathetic nervous activity mentioned previously also inhibits the release of appetite-suppressing leptin while

"Catching Up" on Sleep: Myth or Reality?

Does it help if you're able to sleep longer on some nights of the week? The evidence is mixed. A study by Australian researchers at the University of Sydney looked at nineteen young men who habitually got about six hours of sleep on work nights, then slept in on the weekends. When they had their sleep restricted for several nights in the lab and then were allowed to sleep ten hours a night for three consecutive nights, their insulin sensitivity rebounded significantly compared to their sleep-restricted state.

On the other hand, lack of sleep on weeknights appears to take a long-term toll: A U.S. study published in 2010 that analyzed data from nearly 1,500 subjects found that over a six-year period, those who slept less than six hours a night during the workweek were almost five times more likely to develop prediabetes compared to those who slept six hours or more.

boosting production of the appetite-stimulating hormone *ghrelin,* which has been found to be higher in people who are sleep deprived. This dual effect may help explain why people who sleep less are also more prone to obesity—the preeminent risk factor for type 2 diabetes. Another possible reason lack of sleep could lead to obesity is that people who are chronically fatigued may be less physically active and may also burn fewer calories at rest. Obesity is also a primary cause of sleep apnea, which can disrupt sleep even further, creating a vicious cycle for many people struggling to control their glucose levels.

- Cytokines, immune system components that promote inflammation, have also been found to increase with as little as one night of reduced sleep. And as I discussed in detail in previous chapters, cytokines and other pro-inflammatory molecules contribute directly to insulin resistance and diabetes risk by blocking the effects of insulin.

- Finally, it's been shown that when people are sleep-deprived, their brains utilize less glucose. Because the brain runs on glucose—consuming up to 60% of the body's glucose supply in a resting state—this leaves significantly more blood glucose for the rest of the body to dispose of. It's also been suggested that by disturbing our natural circadian rhythm, sleeping too little at night may interfere with the natural ebb and flow of the body's insulin production and glucose utilization in other subtle ways.

How to Get a Full Night's Sleep

The population of people who are chronically sleep deprived can be divided into several groups—those who intentionally get less sleep than their body needs, due to the demands of their work, home responsibilities, and lifestyle; those who have difficulty getting to sleep or remaining asleep during the night; and those who may be sleeping a full seven or eight hours, but have poor quality sleep during that time, usually because of sleep-related breathing disorders—the most common one being *sleep apnea.* In this next section, I'll address each of these situations in turn.

Natural Approaches to Getting a Better Night's Sleep

S ome 40 million Americans report that they have ongoing problems either falling or staying asleep, and another 20 million report occasional difficulties in these areas. Sleep experts agree that one of the keys to getting a good night's sleep on a consistent basis is to support your body's natural sleep mechanisms in every possible way by doing the following:

WAKE UP AT THE SAME TIME EACH DAY.

Your sleep is controlled by your daily circadian rhythms. This includes a lowering of your core body temperature at night—a drop essential to sleep, with body temperature reaching its lowest point around 4 a.m.— and the nighttime release of the hormone melatonin, which encourages sleep by inducing drowsiness and triggering the aforementioned drop in body temperature. Waking up at the same every day gives these rhythms a consistent fixed orientation point, ensuring that your sleep pattern stays aligned with these internal rhythms—meaning that you'll fall asleep more reliably at night.

EXPOSE YOUR EYES TO DIRECT SUNLIGHT DURING THE DAY.

Exposing your eyes to sunlight (outdoors, without sunglasses) sends signals to your brain's hypothalamus, the area that regulates your circadian rhythms, thereby reinforcing your wake-sleep cycle. In general, the more your eyes are exposed to light during the day, the more soundly you'll sleep at night. If you live at a latitude that gets little sunlight during the winter, you can achieve the same effect by purchasing the type of light box used to treat seasonal affective disorder, or SAD. You will need a model that gives off at least 10,000 lux (cost: approximately $200–$300).

KEEP YOUR SLEEPING ENVIRONMENT AS DARK AS POSSIBLE.

As noted previously, sufficient melatonin production is important to healthy sleep. The brain secretes melatonin only in darkness, however— and ceases production when exposed to bright light. That's why you should keep your bedroom as dark as possible while sleeping—using light-blocking shades or curtains if necessary and covering any light-emitting electronic devices—and use only a dim light for illumination if you need to get up in the night. It's also a good idea to keep your house lights low and avoid the bright stimulation of television or a computer screen in the hour or two before bedtime. This will allow your natural melatonin production to get underway, enabling you to fall asleep quickly.

KEEP YOUR BEDROOM COMFORTABLY COOL.

A too-warm room can partially blunt the all-important sleep-inducing drop in body temperature that occurs during sleep. On the other hand, you'll help encourage this drop by keeping your bedroom's temperature relatively low and using a blanket to keep yourself warm.

AVOID ALL CAFFEINE AFTER LUNCH.

To make sure this stimulant doesn't affect your ability to fall asleep at night, sleep experts advise taking in no caffeine whatsoever within eight hours of your normal bedtime. That includes not only coffee and tea but also caffeinated soda, energy drinks, and chocolate.

DON'T DRINK ALCOHOL NEAR BEDTIME.

Sleep studies have shown that drinking more than a small amount of alcohol in the evening makes your sleep shallower and less restorative and will also cause you to waken in the night. The more alcohol you consume, the greater these effects. If you tend to wake up in the middle of the night and have trouble falling back to sleep, you should avoid drinking any alcoholic beverages after dinner. If you have trouble falling asleep in the first place, then you may want to skip alcohol with your dinner as well because its irritant effect will be peaking around your bedtime.

TAKE A HOT BATH TWO HOURS BEFORE GOING TO BED.

As noted previously, a drop in your core body temperature during the night is a key part of healthy sleep. By raising your body temperature with a hot bath, you'll trigger a "rebound" drop in body temperature one to two hours later, making it easier to fall asleep.

DON'T NAP.

If you have trouble falling or staying asleep at night, napping during the day will only make the problem worse by decreasing the "sleep pressure" that causes you to nod off at night.

TRY A SLEEP-PROMOTING NATURAL SUPPLEMENT.

There are a number of natural products that can also help promote a good night's sleep. Individual responses tend to vary, but research has shown that melatonin supplements—in either capsule or sublingual lozenge form—as well as chamomile tea, kava kava tea, and valerian can all promote sleep in some people. Another natural sleep enhancer is *gamma-aminobutyric acid (GABA)*, a relaxation-promoting neurotransmitter that is widely available as an over-the-counter supplement. Amazon.com, for example, lists dozens of different GABA manufacturers, selling versions ranging from capsules and powder products to flavored chewable GABA tablets.

Supplements that boost brain levels of the neurotransmitter serotonin may also help. Serotonin deficiency has been linked to depression, anxiety, and other stress-related disorders, and pharmaceutical drugs that boost serotonin levels are among the most widely used types of antidepressant medications. You can also boost serotonin levels by taking *5-hydroxytryptophan (5HTP)*, the substance that the body uses to manufacture the neurotransmitter serotonin. A daily supplement of 5HTP increases the body's serotonin production, promoting relaxation, a sense of well-being, and better resistance to stress. Supplements of the amino acid *tryptophan* can also boost serotonin levels (although foods high in tryptophan, such as bananas, don't contain enough of the amino acid to have any serotonin-boosting effect). Researchers at the University of California, San Francisco, led by Dr. Michael German, have also shown that tryptophan can stimulate the growth of new insulin-producing beta cells in the pancreas, helping to prevent the pancreas failure associated with the onset of full-blown type 2 diabetes.

Note: Because these supplements can cause various side effects in certain individuals, check with your doctor before trying any of them.

Sleep Apnea as a Type 2 Diabetes Risk Factor: Why Snoring Is No Laughing Matter

C ould your snoring be harming your ability to metabolize glucose? The evidence is mounting that moderate to severe obstructive sleep apnea—a condition marked by persistent interruptions in breathing during sleep, which is often accompanied by chronic snoring—is an independent risk factor for diabetes. Because these breath stoppages rouse the sleeper to a near-awake state, making it impossible to stay in deep sleep, sleep apnea prevents people from getting a full, restful night's sleep—even though it often *seems* as if they are logging seven or eight hours in the sack. Sleep apnea also exerts an additional negative effect on the body by causing a brief drop in blood oxygen levels with each breath stoppage, a condition known as hypoxia. (See section: What Is Sleep Apnea?)

Animal studies suggest that these frequent drops in blood oxygen levels have a direct negative effect on the body's ability to metabolize glucose. When mice were exposed to seven hours of "intermittent hypoxia," mimicking the effects of sleep apnea, their insulin sensitivity was measurably reduced.

What the Studies Show

W hen trying to figure out whether sleep apnea is a contributing cause of diabetes, population studies must first account for obesity, because excess weight is both a risk factor for diabetes and one of the main underlying causes of sleep apnea.

- One of the largest such studies, the Sleep Heart Health Study, analyzed data from over 2,600 adults and found that, independent of body weight and waist circumference, those with mild sleep apnea were 1.27 times more likely to have fasting glucose intolerance, as measured by an oral glucose tolerance test, than people with normal sleep-related breathing patterns, and that those with moderate to severe sleep apnea were 1.46 times more likely to have fasting glucose intolerance.

- Looking at the connection in the opposite direction, researchers at the University of Chicago evaluated sixty subjects with type 2 diabetes in a sleep lab and found that 77% had obstructive sleep apnea. The study, which was published in 2010, also found the more severe the apnea was, the higher the subjects' hemoglobin A1C levels were, independent of their body fat levels.

Of course, the fact that these two conditions coexist isn't proof that sleep apnea can actually *cause* prediabetes or diabetes. In recent years, however, prospective studies—studies that follow people over time who don't have type 2 diabetes but who do have potential risk factors for the condition, to see what happens to them—have found evidence that sleep apnea may in fact play a contributing role in the impairment of glucose metabolism.

- Another Swedish study followed more than 2,600 middle-aged men for ten years. It found that those who suffered from habitual snoring—a frequent sign of sleep apnea—at the start of the research project were more than twice as likely to develop type 2 diabetes over the course of the study, independent of their age, body weight, or level of physical activity.

- Similarly, an analysis of 70,000 women who participated in the Nurses' Health Study found that over a ten-year period, those who were regular snorers were twice as likely to develop type 2 diabetes as nonsnorers, independent of their weight, level of physical activity, or family history of diabetes.

- In 2009, Yale researchers published results of a six-year study involving nearly six hundred non-diabetic people suffering from sleep-disordered breathing. Each of the subjects spent a night being evaluated in a sleep laboratory—the gold standard for diagnosing sleep apnea. Overall, those who were confirmed as having apnea were significantly more likely to develop type 2 diabetes over the next several years than those who didn't have apnea. This increased risk was also closely correlated to the severity of the subjects' apnea: The more their apnea disrupted their sleep, the more likely they were to get diabetes.

What Is Sleep Apnea?

I n obstructive sleep apnea, the soft tissue in the throat repeatedly relaxes during sleep to the point where it blocks the upper airway, causing breathing to stop temporarily. Each time this happens, the result is a brief period of hypoxia—a drop in blood oxygen levels that leaves the body temporarily oxygen deprived. Mild apnea, defined as an average of five to fifteen breathing blockages per hour, is quite common, affecting an estimated one in five Americans—putting them at a somewhat increased risk of developing impaired glucose tolerance, as noted in the studies cited previously. About 20 million Americans have moderate to severe sleep apnea, meaning they experience more than fifteen blockages per hour—putting them at significantly increased risk of developing impaired glucose tolerance.

How Do You Know If You Have It?

M any people aren't aware they have sleep apnea because its immediate symptoms aren't noticeable to the person who has it. Those who live with apnea sufferers are often the most likely to notice it, particularly because chronic, loud snoring is a common symptom. Not everyone who snores has apnea, however, and not everyone with apnea snores. If you sleep with someone, ask them to listen to see if they hear you stop breathing during sleep, and if so, how often and for how long at a time. Another option is to set the audio recorder on your smartphone or use a digital or audiotape recorder.

How Sleep Apnea Affects Glucose Metabolism

E xactly how obstructive sleep apnea impairs glucose metabolism remains somewhat speculative, but a number of potential mechanisms have been proposed. Like ordinary sleep deprivation, the frequent drops in blood oxygen levels and the frequent awakenings associated with sleep apnea activate the stress-related sympathetic nervous system and stimulate the release of the stress hormone cortisol—both of which, as noted previously, interfere with insulin's action. There's evidence that apnea decreases levels of insulin-like growth factor I (IGF-I) as well, which has been linked to impaired glucose tolerance. People with sleep apnea have also been found to have elevated levels of pro-inflammatory cytokines, including interleukin-6 (IL-6) and tumor necrosis factor alpha (TNF-α), which interfere with insulin signaling. This inflammatory response, which is independent of obesity, is most likely due to the combined effects of the increased stress response and the lack of deep sleep associated with sleep apnea.

Studies at Johns Hopkins University have found that sleep apnea also appears to impair the pancreas's ability to manufacture insulin—meaning that in addition to requiring the body to produce more insulin, sleep apnea may hasten the day when your pancreas can no longer keep up with your body's increased insulin demand, which is the point at which prediabetes and eventually type 2 diabetes sets in.

The Key Point: Sleep Apnea Treatments Improve Glucose Metabolism

Fortunately, effective treatments for sleep apnea exist—most notably, a method called continuous positive airway pressure (CPAP)—in which pressurized air flow is introduced through a mask that's worn while you sleep. Although the evidence isn't completely clear-cut, several studies have linked the use of CPAP therapy to improved insulin sensitivity and blood glucose control.

In one recent study conducted at McGill University in Canada, thirty-nine adults who had been diagnosed with both sleep apnea and prediabetes were randomly assigned to get two weeks of CPAP treatment in a sleep lab, or two weeks receiving a placebo tablet. All participants were also given an oral glucose tolerance test before and after the two-week study. The researchers found that the subjects who received CPAP therapy had significantly improved insulin sensitivity at the end of the treatment period. Similar studies have shown significant drops in hemoglobin A1C levels following CPAP treatment as well.

Treating Sleep Apnea: CPAP and Beyond

I f you suspect you may have obstructive sleep apnea, talk to your primary care doctor about the possibility of getting tested for the condition. You may want to consult a board-certified sleep disorder specialist prior to testing and treatment. Testing for sleep apnea can be done in a sleep lab, requiring an overnight stay, but home tests are also available. If testing shows that you have sleep apnea, there are a number of different treatment options.

CONTINUOUS POSITIVE AIRWAY PRESSURE (CPAP)

Virtually anyone with sleep apnea can benefit from a CPAP machine. These devices, which typically cost several hundred dollars, feed air from a small air compressor into an airtight mask, increasing the pressure of the air being breathed—which in turn keeps the throat from collapsing. The downside: It can be difficult to tolerate, especially for extended periods of time. One in four people who try the device choose not to use at it all, and many more use it only intermittently. Fortunately, as noted previously, some studies show that using it even for a few days can produce glucose-control benefits that can last for an extended period of time.

VARIATIONS ON CPAP

To increase adherence, a number of CPAP modifications have been introduced, including improved mask designs and humidifier attachments. One of these modified versions, known as *bilevel positive airway pressure,* or BiPAP, increases air pressure as the user inhales then reduces it during exhalation, producing a more natural breathing sensation.

ORAL BITE PLATES

In recent years, a number of oral appliances have been approved for the treatment of mild to moderate sleep apnea. These hinged bite plates pull the jaw forward during sleep. They are usually installed by dentists and may require follow-up visits for adjustment. They work well for mild apnea but are effective for only a portion of those who experience severe apnea.

NASAL DEVICES

Another relatively new treatment is Provent, a disposable device that's attached to the nostrils at night, then thrown away in the morning. Approved several years ago for use in treating sleep apnea, it costs just a few dollars a day and works by restricting the amount of air you breathe out. This keeps the lungs partially inflated, which makes the throat more rigid and less prone to collapse.

IMPLANTED NEUROSTIMULATOR

The implanted neurostimulator is the newest treatment for sleep apnea and was featured in a study published early in 2014 in the *New England Journal of Medicine.* Manufactured by Inspire Medical Systems, it employs a pacemaker-like device implanted in the chest that delivers electrical impulses to a nerve in the jaw, that, when stimulated, causes the tongue to move forward, opening the user's airway. In the *NEJM* study, most of the 126 patients it followed experienced significant reductions in nightly breathing stoppages and drops in oxygen levels. Adherence levels were also high, with almost nine out of ten subjects reporting daily use over the study period.

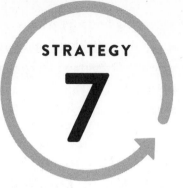

REDUCE STRESS AND MANAGE YOUR MENTAL HEALTH

Acute and chronic stress, along with depression and anxiety—which appear to be caused in large part by chronic stress—have all been found to increase insulin resistance and significantly increase risk for developing prediabetes and type 2 diabetes. By understanding, identifying, and addressing sources of stress, and by taking steps to treat any depression or anxiety you may be experiencing, you will increase your insulin sensitivity, improve your body's ability to metabolize glucose, and reduce your risk of developing type 2 diabetes.

C ould your state of mind or stress level be placing you at greater risk for developing insulin resistance and type 2 diabetes? This link has been suggested for centuries, dating all the way back to the famous seventeenth-century English physician Thomas Willis, who invented the term *diabetes mellitus*—the official medical term for diabetes. "Sadness, or long sorrow, as likewise convulsions, and other depressions and disorders of the animal spirits, are used to generate or foment this morbid disposition," wrote Dr. Willis.

Today, there is a growing body of evidence suggesting that this 350-year-old observation had merit and that both acute and chronic stress, as well as depression and persistent anxiety, can all contribute to impaired glucose metabolism and increase your risk for both prediabetes and type 2 diabetes.

What the Studies Show Regarding Acute and Chronic Stress and Impaired Glucose Metabolism

The fact that acute physical or mental stress can lead to impaired glucose metabolism is well known. People without diabetes who are admitted to acute-care facilities such as in intensive cardiac care units frequently have elevated glucose levels similar to those that someone with diabetes would have. After their acute illness is over, these high glucose levels will often subside. Acute mental stress appears to have a similar effect. Using data obtained before and during the eight-day conflict in the Gaza Strip in 2012, for example, Israeli researchers concluded that exposure to a single intense episode of emotional trauma led to significantly higher glucose levels among hospital admittees.

When stress persists for an extended period of time—a condition known as chronic stress—this metabolic impairment can evolve into a serious risk factor for type 2 diabetes. A number of studies have linked various types of chronic stress to increased prevalence of both insulin resistance and type 2 diabetes. In a Dutch study published in 2000, researchers gave more than 2,200 subjects with no previous history of diabetes a questionnaire inquiring about the number of major stressful life events they had experienced over the preceding five years. Events falling under this category included serious, long-lasting illness or other problems involving a child or partner; the death of a child, partner, relative, or friend; the end of an important relationship; moving from a house; significant financial problems; and work-related issues such as retirement, a forced job change, or serious or long-lasting problems at work.

The investigators then gave each of the subjects an oral glucose test, which showed that 5% of the subjects had previously undetected diabetes.

Comparing the questionnaire results of the diabetes group with the rest of the study population, they found that, after adjusting for age and gender, those who had experienced at least one stressful event over the past five years were 1.2 times more likely to be in the diabetes group than those who had experienced no stressful events. They also found that those who had experienced three or more stressful events during that time period were 1.6 times more likely to have previously undiagnosed type 2 diabetes than those who reported less than three stressful events.

The link between stress and diabetes appears to stretch back all the way to childhood. Another study, published in 2004, looked at data on nearly six thousand people from the National Comorbidity Survey—the first large-scale survey of mental health ever conducted in the United States. In this study, researchers interviewed a large cohort of people in the early 1990s, then interviewed them again ten years later. After adjusting for age, gender, race, and other factors, the researchers found that study subjects who had a self-reported history of childhood neglect were 2.2 times more likely to have been diagnosed with type 2 diabetes than those without such a history. This association was even stronger among women, who were 4.6 times more likely to have diabetes if they reported being neglected as children.

Symptoms of Chronic Stress

Because chronic stress is typically caused by psychological pressures that produce indirect symptoms, people are often unaware that they're being affected by it. You could be suffering from chronic stress if you're experiencing any of the following on a regular basis:

- Unexplained fatigue
- Insomnia
- Difficulty concentrating or forgetfulness
- Irritability
- Nervousness or anxiety
- Anger for no clear reason
- Persistent or intermittent chest pains
- Recurring headaches, backaches, or muscle pain
- Gastrointestinal problems
- Feelings of sadness or depression
- Restlessness or an inability to relax
- Compulsive eating
- Drinking alcohol to excess

Inside Joslin: Studying How Diabetes Affects Brain Function

Led by Dr. Alan Jacobsen, our past chief of psychiatry, and Dr. Gail Musen, assistant professor at Joslin Laboratories, Joslin researchers have been uncovering some fascinating evidence regarding how diabetes affects the brain in ways that might potentially increase the risk of depression. One of the findings of Drs. Jacobsen and Musen is that in people with type 1 diabetes, the prefrontal cortex of the brain (an area that helps regulate emotion) is less dense and responsive compared to the brains of non-diabetics. Another recent Joslin research project showed that high blood sugar levels in type 1 diabetics can cause abnormally high levels of glutamate—a neurotransmitter thought to contribute to depression—to form in this same brain region.

Prospective studies—in which researchers do a baseline evaluation of a group of subjects, then follow them over time to see what happens to them—have found similar connections. In a landmark study published in 2007, Finnish and U.S. researchers identified more than five hundred middle-aged women with no signs of metabolic syndrome—a condition that can include elevated fasting blood glucose and is also associated with increased diabetes risk—and followed them for an average of fifteen years. They found that those women who reported feeling frequently and intensely angry, tensed, or stressed at the start of the study were significantly more likely to develop metabolic syndrome over that time.

Even more striking, a Japanese study, published in 2009, followed more than 55,000 subjects for ten years and found that men with a high stress level were 1.36 times more likely to develop type 2 diabetes over that time, while highly stressed women were 1.22 times more likely to be diagnosed with type 2 diabetes during that same period.

Perhaps most important of all, from *The Diabetes Reset* perspective, is the fact that stress can help accelerate the progression of prediabetes to diabetes in a relatively short period of time. Another Japanese study, published in 2008, followed 128 middle-aged men who had either impaired fasting glucose or impaired glucose tolerance. Over a three-year period, more than one fourth of this group went on to develop type

2 diabetes. The study found that subjects who scored highest on a questionnaire evaluating their stress levels at the start of the study were almost four times as likely to be among those diagnosed with diabetes.

Another interesting study linking chronic stress to increased risk of diabetes comes from the Kohala Health Research Project, which examined the risk of diabetes in Native Hawaiians. They made the intriguing discovery that Native Hawaiians who lived a traditional lifestyle have twice the risk of developing type 2 diabetes as those who have assimilated into the mainstream culture. The researchers concluded that this heightened risk of type 2 diabetes for native Hawaiians living in a traditional mode could not be attributed to any of the usual risk factors of diabetes—suggesting that the main contributing factor was chronic stress derived from the constant challenge of maintaining their traditional lifestyle and values in the midst of Western culture, including trying to sustain their language and traditional religious practices.

Depression and Impaired Glucose Metabolism

It has been thought for many years that having diabetes—either type 1 or type 2—leaves people more prone to developing depression. Indeed, both the American Diabetes Association and our own Joslin website mention studies showing that people with diabetes are more likely to become depressed than people without diabetes. At present, however, the notion that diabetes directly causes depression is open to debate. Earlier studies linking the two conditions were virtually all retrospective, meaning the researchers asked people to think back in time and recall the progression of their diabetes and depression—an approach that is not very reliable in terms of analyzing which condition preceded the other. As you'll see next, some recent large-scale prospective studies—in which people were followed over time to see what happened to them—have not been able to find compelling evidence that diabetes causes depression. As you'll also see, however, these studies did find strong evidence for a causal relationship in the other direction.

This doesn't mean that diabetes can't affect people's mental and emotional well-being. Researchers at the Joslin Diabetes Center have been making some important discoveries about diabetes' effect on the brain, which could theoretically support a biological link between diabetes and increased depression risk. (See box on page 184: Inside Joslin: Studying How Diabetes Affects Brain Function.) But again, this relationship hasn't been borne out in large-scale prospective studies.

The bottom line: As you'll see in the pages that follow, the evidence is quite strong that depression causes an increased risk of diabetes—but there is not much evidence to support the notion that diabetes directly contributes to depression risk.

The first meta-analysis to establish that depression increases risk for developing type 2 diabetes was published by a research team from the Netherlands in 2006. The research team looked only at data from studies that had recruited subjects with no diagnosable diabetes at the time they were enrolled and then performed baseline evaluations of these subjects for both depression and blood glucose metabolism, after which the studies followed the subjects for an extended period of time. After doing a statistical analysis of the nine studies that met their criteria, the researchers found that being depressed increased a person's long-term risk of developing type 2 diabetes by 7%.

Two years later, researchers at Johns Hopkins University and the University of Michigan collaborated on an even more extensive meta-analysis. The goal of their study was to explore the bidirectional relationship between depression and diabetes—looking at how depression affects risk of diabetes as well as how diabetes impacts depression risk. For the first arm of the project, the researchers analyzed thirteen studies that were designed to evaluate whether depression leads to increased diabetes risk, involving nearly seven thousand subjects in all. Their analysis found that depression was associated with a 60% increased risk of developing type 2 diabetes over time.

To evaluate the relationship in the other direction—looking for an indication that having diabetes put someone at greater risk for developing depression—the researchers looked at an additional seven studies designed to study the risk of depression in diabetics. Their analysis of this group of projects, which had followed a total of more than 6,400 people over an extended period, found that having type 2 diabetes increased the relative risk of becoming clinically depressed by 1.15 times.

ANXIETY AND DIABETES RISK

Finally, there is also evidence that persistent feelings of anxiety may also increase risk for type 2 diabetes—and that the combination of anxiety and depression may boost diabetes risk even more. A large Norwegian study of 37,000 men and women, which involved an initial assessment and a follow-up evaluation ten years later, found that subjects who reported significant anxiety or depression at the start of the study were 1.5 times more likely to develop type 2 diabetes over the next decade than people who didn't have either condition and that those suffering from both conditions had a 1.8 times greater risk of eventually being diagnosed with diabetes.

How Stress, Depression, and Anxiety Affect Glucose Metabolism

Despite the evidence outlined in the preceding section linking stress to diabetes risk, we don't yet have a clear understanding of the underlying connection between chronic stress and mood disorders and impaired glucose metabolism. Some possible theories for this connection have been offered, however. These generally focus on the impact of two different groups of factors: how stress, depression, and anxiety impact people's behavior, and the effects these conditions have on body chemistry.

THE BEHAVIORAL IMPACT OF DEPRESSION

One potential reason that stress and mood disorders could increase diabetes risk is that when people are under chronic stress or suffering from depression or anxiety, they are more likely to overeat, eat foods high in fat and sugar, and be physically inactive—all behaviors that increase risk of obesity, insulin resistance, and type 2 diabetes.

There is considerable evidence to support this idea. Animal studies have shown a direct connection between chronic stress and a heightened affinity for "comfort food" that is high in fat and sugar. (See section: Self-Medicating with Fat and Sugar: The Stress–Comfort Food Link). And a meta-analysis of sixteen human studies, published in 2008, concluded that "after controlling for potential confounding variables, depressed

Is Your Job Giving You Diabetes?

If you have a stressful job and you've either been diagnosed with prediabetes or type 2 diabetes or have risk factors for these conditions, you may want to consider making a change. A number of studies have found that work-related stress has a significant impact on your body's metabolic health. In particular, jobs that combine heavy work demands with a limited control over decision making appear to increase people's risk for developing type 2 diabetes.

In one research paper published in 2006, researchers analyzed data from a prospective study that followed more than ten thousand British civil servants for an average of fourteen years. Over that time, their work stress was measured at four different points using the iso-strain model, which identifies stressful jobs as those that are highly demanding and give workers little or no latitude in terms of decision making—with an even higher amount of stress assigned to jobs that are also isolated, offering no support from coworkers or supervisors. The researchers found a direct dose response between the amount of work stress experienced by subjects and their risk of developing metabolic syndrome—a cluster of symptoms that includes insulin resistance and is a leading risk factor for type 2 diabetes. Those who reported high work stress at least three times during the study were nearly twice as likely to be diagnosed with metabolic syndrome as those with no exposure to work stress.

These findings were confirmed by a recent Swedish study that followed 5,400 women and men with no history of impaired glucose tolerance for about a decade. Those who ranked in the highest third in terms of work demands and the lowest third in terms of their freedom to decide how to perform their work were 1.6 times more likely to develop type 2 diabetes after all other factors were accounted for, including family history of diabetes, BMI, physical activity level, and other sources of psychological distress. Women were particularly affected by this type of job stress, with diabetes risk more than quadrupling for those with high job demands and low decision-making latitude. At the same time, those with high job demands who also had a high level of freedom in making decisions actually saw benefits from their work situation: Their risk of developing diabetes was half that of the study population as a whole.

compared to nondepressed people were at significantly higher risk for developing obesity." Another paper, published in 2009, analyzed a research study that followed 4,300 middle-aged British civil servants—none of whom were obese at the start of the study—for nineteen years. It found that those with the highest rate of anxiety, depression, and other common mental disorders were the most likely to become obese over the course of that study.

Depression also appears to reduce people's physical activity levels. A meta-analysis of eleven studies, published in the journal *General Hospital Psychiatry* in 2009, concluded that over time, "Depression may be a significant risk factor for development of sedentary lifestyle or decreased level of physical exercise." As I discussed in Strategy Chapter 3, physical inactivity is both a risk factor for insulin resistance in and of itself, and it can also contribute to weight gain.

BIOLOGICAL LINKS BETWEEN STRESS AND MOOD DISORDERS AND DIABETES RISK

Although stress is commonly thought of as a mental and emotional issue, it actually has a measurable effect on a person's body chemistry. Short-term stress—being faced with an immediate physical or psychological threat, such as a near-accident while driving or a confrontation with an angry coworker—causes your sympathetic "fight or flight" nervous system to switch on, flooding your body with the hormones epinephrine (adrenaline) and norepinephrine. These biochemicals immediately trigger a wide range of physical responses, including an increase in heart rate, sweating, and constriction of the blood vessels. This acute stress response also causes the liver to metabolize some of its glycogen—the form in which glucose is stored in the body—into glucose to supply your muscles with ready energy for dealing with whatever emergency is on hand. The result is a temporary spike in blood glucose levels.

As powerful as this stress response is, however, it tends to be short-lived. For someone concerned about improving his or her insulin sensitivity and preventing or reversing prediabetes or type 2 diabetes, chronic stress is a much more dangerous factor. This type of stress, defined as ongoing emotional distress that can't be controlled—when someone is a daily caregiver to a very ill relative, for example—results in prolonged elevation of another set of stress hormones, known as glucocorticoids, which are regulated by a brain network known as the hypothalamic-pituitary-adrenal (HPA) axis. There is intriguing evidence that chronic stimulation of this network, which occurs in chronic stress, anxiety, and depression, boosts levels of abdominal fat—the type of fat that interferes the most with insulin sensitivity. In a 2010 publication, for example, researchers looked at data from the Coronary Artery Risk Development in Young Adults Study, which assessed more than five thousand young adults at regular five-year intervals, and found that those who scored highest on a survey evaluating depression also gained the most abdominal fat over the course of the study.

In humans, the most prevalent of these chronic stress hormones is cortisol. One of cortisol's properties is to help regulate blood glucose levels, making sure they don't dip too low. It does this by directly blocking the action of insulin. Studies have found that increased blood cortisol levels reduce the ability of muscle and fat cells to take up blood glucose and also blunt insulin's glucose-suppressing effects in the liver, thereby encouraging the liver to manufacture more glucose than it otherwise would. There is even evidence that cortisol's insulin resistance–causing effects (and the increase in insulin production this leads to) may inhibit the ability of the pancreas to produce insulin in a regulated manner.

All of us have cortisol circulating in our body constantly, with levels peaking just before we wake up in the morning and then declining throughout the day. When cortisol levels are chronically elevated, however, as they are in people suffering from chronic stress, depression, and anxiety, this can contribute to insulin resistance. In animal studies, for example, lab rats that were administered glucocorticoids in utero went on to develop insulin resistance as mature rats. A number of studies have also shown an association between elevated cortisol and insulin resistance in people. In a 1998 British study of 370 men ages sixty to seventy, those with the highest blood cortisol levels in the morning after fasting overnight had the highest blood glucose levels upon awakening as well. When they were subsequently given an oral glucose tolerance test, the researchers found that this group also had higher insulin resistance than the other men in the study.

A clear example of high levels of cortisol leading to insulin resistance and diabetes can be found in people suffering from Cushing's syndrome, a disease in which cortisol levels are chronically elevated due to tumors or overuse of steroid medications. Most people with Cushing's syndrome are insulin resistant and 20% go on to develop diabetes. (Note: Because steroid medications are used to reduce inflammation, they can actually benefit glucose metabolism in the short run—but when used chronically, they can actually cause insulin resistance and diabetes.)

Chronic stress also results in increased levels of pro-inflammatory cytokines—the same inflammation-producing chemicals that are produced by enlarged fat stores and other stressed body tissues, which have been shown to interfere with insulin signaling. And finally, anxiety, chronic stress, and depression all tend to result in poor-quality sleep—which, as we saw in Strategy Chapter 6, also reduces insulin sensitivity and increases risk for type 2 diabetes.

Chronic Stress and Cortisol: A Vicious Cycle

Have you ever gone through a period of extended stress—a particularly demanding stretch of work, for example—and found yourself getting short-tempered over things you ordinarily wouldn't be bothered by? What you were experiencing was the vicious cycle of chronic stress: Animal studies have clearly demonstrated that when a lab animal is chronically stressed, its brain reacts more strongly to new sources of stress as well, producing greater amounts of cortisol than the brain of an animal that is not chronically stressed. In other words, chronic stress is not only damaging in and of itself—it also leaves you more vulnerable to the effects of any other stresses you may encounter.

Self-Medicating with Fat and Sugar:
The Stress–Comfort Food Link

When the stress starts to build at home or on the job, do you find yourself automatically reaching for a cookie or a bag of potato chips? What's actually happening, according to recent research findings, is that your body is attempting to self-medicate by reducing the stress reaction in your brain. In the past few years, a number of fascinating studies have produced evidence suggesting that we may be hardwired to seek out high-fat, high-sugar foods when we're exposed to chronic stress.

Animal studies have shown that when high levels of cortisol are produced by exposure to stress while insulin levels are also elevated (as they are in people with insulin resistance), this leads to an increased appetite for high-fat foods. These studies have also found that eating food of this type actually reduces the stress-related activation of the brain's HPA region by stimulating the pleasure-oriented part of that region. Other animal studies have found that stress experienced as a newborn can actually create a lifelong preference for high-fat, high-sugar food over regular animal chow.

These responses have been echoed in human studies showing that stress increases people's affinity for high-fat or high-sugar "comfort foods." Eating high-fat food also appears to reduce the impact of stress in another, longer-term way, by preferentially encouraging the growth of abdominal fat. For reasons that have not yet been discovered, abdominal fat is associated with reduced activation of the brain's stress response—meaning that, although this type of body fat is clearly bad for our physical health, it appears to provide a certain amount of emotional comfort when we're under stress.

How to Manage Stress and Relieve Depression and Anxiety

The simplest approach to relieving chronic stress, of course, is to simply avoid whatever is causing it. As we all know, however, this can be quite difficult and often impossible. Obviously, there are certain stresses that can't be avoided—just as there's nothing you can do to change stress-ful events in your past. The illness or death of a loved one, a difficult job, or financial pressures are things we can't just walk away from.

It is possible, however, to change how we *react* to stressors, both past and present, to at least some degree. Stress management techniques typically aim to do this either by modifying your physiological response to stress or altering the way you perceive stress on an intellectual or emotional level. There are a variety of proven approaches to manag-ing stress, which, when implemented correctly—either individually or in concert—can go a long way toward neutralizing the mental or physi-ological effects of stress.

These approaches fall into four general categories:

- Making changes in your daily life that can help you handle, defuse, or sidestep stress more effectively

- Targeted stress-reduction techniques, designed to switch off the body's sympathetic (fight or flight) nervous system

- Psychotherapeutic approaches that aim to change a person's psy-chological response to whatever stresses he or she is experiencing

- Medications or supplements that will help counter the physiologi-cal results of stress

Making Stress-Reducing Changes in Your Daily Life

When feeling hemmed in by stress, it's easy to forget that you do have options. By exploring these options, you'll not only feel bet-ter at the moment, but you'll also remind yourself that you are not as trapped as you think.

TAKE TIME FOR YOURSELF

It may sound obvious, but simply taking time out for yourself can be immensely helpful, at least in the near term, when dealing with ongo-ing stress. Heading to the movies, taking a short vacation, or even just relaxing in a bath can help clear your head and may even point the way toward some positive next steps you can take.

EMBRACE A FAVORITE PASTIME

You probably have a hobby or pastime you find engrossing. Immersing yourself in your own favorite activity will help stimulate your parasympathetic nervous system—the network that counters your fight or flight mechanism—and will also get you into what psychologists call a "flow state," in which you are at peace with your environment.

EXERCISE

I've already discussed how exercise directly improves glucose metabolism. But from swimming or cycling to golf or tennis, research has shown that sustained physical activity also has a powerful stress-reducing effect. This may be due in part to the release of endorphins—the brain's natural pain-relieving chemicals—that takes place during physical activity. Exercise also has a meditative element, which can help induce the body's natural relaxation response, and enhances mood as well. It also improves the quality of sleep, which is often disturbed by chronic stress.

SEEK OUT SOCIAL SUPPORT

Research has shown that a well-developed social support network of family, friends, and colleagues enhances psychological and physical health even in the best of times. When you're under stress, this social support becomes even more critical. Not only has it been shown to directly relieve stress, but it also helps people adjust more readily to stressful situations they can't avoid. A number of factors appear to be involved in the positive benefits of social support, including the chance to express negative feelings; enhanced feelings of self-efficacy from the positive feedback of others; the increased availability of helpful information and logistical support; and the positive psychological effects of emotional connection and involvement with others.

Although social support can, and often does, come from many different sources on an informal basis, you may also want to connect with more formalized support networks such as a spiritual group, a community-based social organization, a professionally led peer support group, or a targeted support service such as those developed to assist people who have a chronic or disabling illness or are caring for a loved one with a condition of this type. As noted earlier, connecting with work colleagues can be especially important if you have a demanding yet isolating job, which experts have identified as being particularly stressful.

Stress-Reduction Techniques

A variety of specific techniques have been proven effective at countering the mental and physiological effects of stress by activating the parasympathetic nervous system, which works in opposition to the sympathetic nervous system's fight or flight mechanism.

MEDITATIVE BREATHING

By focusing on slow, regular breathing while also keeping your mind concentrated on a sound or image that is non–stress related, you can switch on your parasympathetic system and feel a sense of calm. This technique has been in use for centuries, and plays a central role in many spiritual practices.

WHAT TO DO. Find a quiet place where you can sit comfortably. Set a timer to go off after fifteen or twenty minutes, so you won't need to check the clock. Close your eyes and concentrate for a minute or two on relaxing your muscles completely. Next, begin breathing in slowly through your nose, taking several seconds to complete your inhalation, then exhale slowly in the same way. As you get accustomed to this pattern, begin silently repeating a single word, sound, or short phrase with each in-breath and out-breath. This mantra should be something you find soothing and that has no special meaning to you. The idea is not to associate that word or sound with anything in particular. Common mantras include *one, peace, calm mind,* and *letting go.* The classic Buddhist mantra, of course, is *om*—a syllable that is thought to be the sound of the universe.

Continue breathing in and out slowly with your eyes closed, focusing on your mantra. As your mind wanders to other topics, simply guide it back in a nonjudgmental way to your mantra. Try to do this for fifteen to twenty minutes at a time, several days a week or more.

PROGRESSIVE MUSCLE RELAXATION

This relaxation technique, also known as PMR, involves tensing and then relaxing each part of the body in turn. An abbreviated version of PMR is sometimes used prior to meditation. Studies have shown this approach is effective at reducing both stress and anxiety. CDs and free downloads that can guide you through the process are widely available.

WHAT TO DO. Start by sitting comfortably or lying down. PMR can be done with your eyes open or closed. Each muscle group should be tensed hard but without straining for five to ten seconds, then relaxed completely. Then wait ten seconds or more before tensing the next muscle group. You can start with any body part you wish, but move completely through that body area before going to the next one. Sample progression: feet, lower legs, thighs, buttocks, abdomen, back, chest, shoulders, hands, forearms, upper arms, neck, mouth and jaw, eyes, forehead. When you're finished, remain still for several minutes, experiencing the feeling of relaxation in all the muscles of your body. A complete session will typically take about twenty minutes.

MINDFULNESS-BASED STRESS REDUCTION

Also known as MBSR, this is another type of meditative approach to reducing stress and anxiety. It was developed by Dr. Jon Kabat-Zinn, a molecular biologist by training who is also a student of Zen Buddhism, and it is based on the ancient Buddhist practice of mindfulness. The Stress Reduction Clinic founded by Dr. Kabat-Zinn at the University of Massachusetts pioneered the use of mindfulness as a way of coping with chronic pain and other conditions. Today, it's widely used as an adjunct therapy to medical treatments, particularly as a method of pain management, and is also coming into increasing use as a treatment for post-traumatic stress disorder (PTSD).

Instead of trying to steer the mind away from thoughts associated with stress, as other forms of meditation do, mindfulness training encourages people to be "in the moment" and to pay close attention to the feelings or sensations that are giving rise to their stress but in an open, nonjudgmental way. It is frequently described as getting off "auto pilot" and living more fully in the present, but this increased focus also involves becoming more aware of your reactions to the world around you. The idea is that by tapping into a preexisting state of calm, you can gain control over your responses to what were perceived as sources of stress, thereby reducing or eliminating the stress. MBSR may also incorporate yoga poses to promote physical relaxation.

WHAT TO DO. Although most proponents of mindful meditation recommend getting formal training in how to practice it, here are some ways you can explore this approach right now:

- Sit quietly and observe your breath, listening to it and feeling the sensation as you inhale and exhale. Don't try to control your breathing: Simply let the air move in and out of your body naturally, as you concentrate all of your attention on it. This focus on your breath can be used as a touchstone for mindfulness practice. By taking a moment to observe your breath in this way before any new activity or encounter, you can quickly calm and center yourself.

- Spend a few minutes doing a full mental scan of your body, starting with your feet and moving up your body. When you notice a spot of tension, discomfort, or pain, linger on that place with your mind, focusing on the sensation itself—what it actually feels like and where it begins and ends.

- Sit quietly for an extended period of time observing your own thoughts. If a stressful thought arises—some task that needs to be done or a relationship or situation that is troubling you—simply note that thought and any accompanying emotions without judgment, then continue to focus on the present moment as you watch your thoughts come and go.

BIOFEEDBACK

This is another potentially powerful tool for managing your physical and mental response to stress. In general, the term refers to any system of monitoring physiologic reactions that you ordinarily aren't aware of and using this feedback to modify how you respond to various stimuli. One

simple form of biofeedback for stress management is simply to monitor your pulse rate. As you become calmer, your pulse rate will become
slower. If you sit or lie quietly and check the pulse in one wrist with the
first two fingertips of the opposite hand, over time you'll find that you
can actually get your pulse rate to slow down by relaxing, breathing in a
slow, even fashion, and thinking calming thoughts.

Another simple biofeedback approach is to look at your reflection
in the mirror and concentrate on relaxing your facial muscles. A more
sophisticated type of biofeedback for stress reduction involves a galvanic skin response monitor. This device measures the conductivity
of your skin, which becomes greater as you sweat more at rest—which
happens when your sympathetic nervous system is activated by stress.
It typically involves a monitoring element that slips over the user's finger and is connected to an electrical receiver. Some versions emit a tone
calibrated to the conductivity level, with the tone dropping lower as you
become calmer. Reliable galvanic skin response devices are available at
prices beginning around $70.

The most widely used forms of biofeedback stress reduction in a
clinical setting involve the use of an electromyograph (EMG) or elec-
troencephalograph (EEG).

- An EMG device measures the tension in a targeted muscle group
  and helps the user learn to either relax or contract those muscles.
  This approach may be used to treat chronic pain, anxiety, high blood
  pressure, and incontinence, among other disorders.

- An EEG device measures brain wave activity, using electrodes that are
  taped to the scalp. EEG stress reduction therapy typically focuses on
  teaching the user to generate alpha waves—the relatively slow wave
  patterns associated with meditative calm. Conditions treated with
  this approach include anxiety disorders, depression, and addiction.

Many academic medical centers now have biofeedback facilities, and
freestanding biofeedback practices can also be found throughout the U.S.
If you decide to try biofeedback therapy, be sure to go to a trained prac-
titioner certified by the Biofeedback Certification Institute of America.

YOGA

The stress-reducing effects of yoga have been known for centuries and have also been validated by numerous research studies. With its emphasis on breathing, calm awareness, and relaxation of the muscles, yoga has elements in common with many other stress-reduction techniques and is often used as a component of mindfulness-based stress-reduction. It has powerful benefits on its own as well: In one German study, for example, two dozen emotionally distressed women who attended twice-weekly yoga classes for three months saw significant improvement in measures of anxiety, depression, and perceived stress. It has also been found to help people suffering from post-traumatic stress disorder. Studies suggest that you'll get the best results by attending a sixty- to ninety-minute class at least once a week for several months.

SELF-HYPNOSIS

Self-hypnosis can be an effective stress-management tool as well: By promoting a state of relaxation and reinforcing an attitude of calm acceptance on the subconscious level, you can modify your conscious response to stress. Studies have found it to be effective in managing various types of pain as well as anxiety- and stress-related disorders.

WHAT TO DO. Choose a quiet place and set aside twenty to thirty minutes. Begin by focusing on a positive phrase that describes the thought or behavior you want to achieve in the self-hypnosis session. For example, you might say to yourself: "I am accomplishing my work in a calm, efficient manner" or "My pain is lessening." Next, sit quietly and spend several minutes breathing slowly and deeply, allowing a feeling of relaxation to spread throughout your body. When you are fully relaxed, envision yourself passing slowly into a new realm. Different images can be employed for this. Possibilities include:

- Rowing slowly across a lake and then climbing up a ladder on the far side to a high plateau

- Descending a stairway step by step into a cool space or a body of water

- Walking down a long corridor to reach a door at the far side
- Going farther and farther into a forest until you reach a distant clearing

As you move through this passage toward whatever your destination is, feel yourself entering an ever-deeper state of relaxation. Once you reach your destination, you'll be ready to begin giving yourself your chosen hypnotic suggestion. Imagine yourself walking through your new-found space, populating it with whatever images you want. At the same time, begin repeating to yourself the phrase you selected at the start of the session. Continue repeating this phrase for as long as you want, as your imagination leads through your envisioned world.

When you have finished repeating your chosen phrase, make your journey in reverse, gradually bringing yourself out of your state of deep relaxation as you do. Once you are back in your normal conscious state, continue to sit and breathe in a relaxed fashion for several minutes longer.

Stress-Reduction Psychotherapy

For more severe chronic stress, structured psychotherapy can be an effective tool for reframing thoughts and behavior. Here are some of the most common psychotherapeutic approaches used for stress reduction:

COGNITIVE-BEHAVIORAL THERAPY (CBT)

This form of targeted, short-term therapy has come into wide use for anxiety- and stress-related disorders as well as depression. In this approach, the therapist encourages the client to examine negative thinking patterns linked to various anxieties and stresses and to replace unrealistic, overblown, or irrational fears and concerns—such as catastrophic thinking (imagining the worst possible outcome), overemphasizing the negative aspect of things, overpersonalizing (connecting any problem to a personal shortcoming—for example, consistently assigning other people's upset feelings to the fact that you failed them somehow), or viewing issues as totally black and white—with a more realistic assessment of the threats posed by the stressful situation. This cognitive technique is supplemented by behavioral methods such as positive self-talk, goal setting, and the development of coping skills.

Research suggests that a limited course of CBT can be highly effective at alleviating chronic stress and stress-related disorders. A 2013 publication reported that twelve sessions of CBT not only improved symptoms in subjects suffering from post-traumatic stress disorder but also resulted in enlargement in the hippocampus region of their brains, which has been shown to shrink as a result of traumatic stress. Similarly, a review of multiple meta-analyses published in 2010 concluded that CBT had been shown to be effective across a range of anxiety disorders. It has also been found to be effective for both moderate and severe depression, particularly when combined with pharmacologic therapy.

To find a certified cognitive-behavioral therapist near you, visit the website of the National Association of Cognitive-Behavioral Therapists at nacbt.org.

PSYCHODYNAMIC THERAPY

In this approach, commonly referred to as talk therapy, the therapist encourages the client to explore his or her feelings of stress, anxiety, sadness, or depression and connect them to conflicts in current and past relationships. Although it typically involves a longer course of treatment than CBT—up to a year, in many cases—there is a large body of evidence attesting to its effectiveness. A 2010 review paper looked at eight different meta-analyses of the effectiveness of psychodynamic therapy, encompassing 160 studies in all, and concluded that this therapeutic approach showed substantial benefits for a wide range of psychological conditions, including anxiety, panic disorders, stress-related physical problems, and depression.

Seeking Medical Care for Depression and Anxiety

Although all of the therapeutic techniques described in this chapter can be effective in certain cases, there are also times when a psychological or emotional condition requires professional medical care and perhaps medication as well. If you find you have persistent feelings of sadness or hopelessness that are interfering with your sleeping or eating or making it difficult to pursue or enjoy your normal activities, you should discuss these symptoms with your doctor immediately. You may be suffering from clinical depression, which typically responds best to a combination of psychotherapy and antidepressant medication.

Similarly, if you are experiencing worries, recurring fears, or panic attacks that are interfering with your daily life, you should seek professional medical care for an anxiety disorder. There are a number of anti-anxiety medications and other targeted medical therapies that are very effective for treating such disorders.

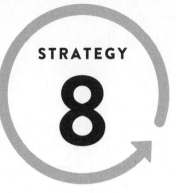

BOOST YOUR OWN NATURAL ANTIOXIDANTS

Oxidative stress, caused by excessive amounts of volatile molecules called "reactive oxygen species" (ROS) in the tissues of the body, has been linked to dysfunction in mitochondria, the tiny energy factories that power every cell in your body. This dysfunction in turn has been directly linked to the development of insulin resistance. Oxidative stress can also damage the beta cells of the pancreas and contributes to many of the complications caused by elevated glucose levels when type 1 or type 2 diabetes is poorly controlled. For all of these reasons, people with glucose metabolism problems can benefit significantly from activating the body's natural antioxidants by ingesting foods rich in "Phase 2 antioxidants," which stimulate the body's natural production of antioxidants on the cellular level.

J ust about everyone has heard about how toxic oxygen molecules, including those known as "free radicals," can damage our bodies and how antioxidants are the secret to neutralizing these nasty little molecules. This has led to the popular belief that taking hefty doses of specific nutrients with antioxidant properties—most notably, vitamin E and vitamin C—is the key to good health. As you'll learn in this chapter, however, the story of oxidative damage and antioxidants isn't so simple. This point was demonstrated vividly in a recent study coauthored by Dr. C. Ronald Kahn, a senior investigator and head of the Integrative Physiology and Metabolism Department at Joslin.

Dr. Kahn and his research colleagues were interested in learning more about the process by which exercise reduces insulin resistance. We know that this process occurs at least in part because the muscle contractions involved in exercise lead to increased energy production by the

The Limited Benefits of Vitamins E and C

A recent Joslin study (see page 205) appears to show vitamin E and vitamin C actively interfering with the diabetes-fighting benefits of exercise. A number of other research projects have also looked at whether supplements of these antioxidant vitamins are a help or a hindrance to preventing or controlling type 2 diabetes. As in Dr. Kahn's experiment, their evidence suggests these vitamins do little good and may actually be harmful—most likely because these vitamins scavenge ROS that are already in circulation throughout the body, while the oxidative stress that causes insulin resistance occurs on the cellular level, where your body's natural antioxidants (which are triggered by Phase 2 antioxidants) exert a much more powerful effect.

- A 2011 meta-analysis of the glucose-control effects of vitamin E, a potent antioxidant, found that only people with prior vitamin E deficiencies or poorly controlled diabetes benefited from taking the vitamin, whereas the general pool of type 2 diabetic subjects showed no improvement in glycemic control from vitamin E supplements.

- A 2008 analysis of data from a large-scale prospective European study conducted in the 1990s found that increased blood levels of vitamin C were associated with reduced risk of developing type 2 diabetes. These high levels of vitamin C were linked to eating more fruits and vegetables, however, rather than taking vitamin C supplements. A number of prospective human studies have found that daily supplementation with high doses of Vitamin C had no effect on glycemic control in people with type 2 diabetes. Others have shown modest benefits, such as a recent study in India which found that taking vitamin C along with the diabetes medication metformin produced better glycemic control than taking metformin alone.

muscles' mitochondria, which in turn leads to increased mitochondrial production of "reactive oxygen species" or ROS—that group of potentially toxic oxygen molecules that includes free radicals. We also know that the muscle cells react to these increased quantities of ROS by ramping up production of certain natural antioxidants that help neutralize these ROS after their job is done.

What Dr. Kahn's research group wanted to know was whether taking antioxidant supplements—specifically, vitamin E and vitamin C—interfered with this beneficial process. They found that it did, in a big way: The investigators put two groups of individuals (including some who already exercised regularly and others who didn't) through an intensive month-long exercise program in which each subject worked out for eighty-five minutes per day, five days a week, for a four-week period. One of the groups was also given 400 IU of vitamin E and 1,000 milligrams of vitamin C (the amounts contained in typical vitamin supplements) on a daily basis. Although the nonvitamin group showed the expected exercise-related effects of reduced insulin resistance and increased production of natural antioxidants, the group that got antioxidant supplements did not. In other words, the vitamin supplements not only blocked the diabetes-fighting effects of exercise but also prevented the body's natural antioxidant protection from kicking in!

This is important information because one of the most intriguing new areas of research on insulin resistance and type 2 diabetes involves understanding the effects of ROS. These molecules contain oxygen atoms with extra electrons, which cause them to be highly reactive with other molecules they encounter. As noted previously, one of the best-known types of ROS are free radicals, which are oxygen ions that have lost an electron. But there are other types of ROS as well, including peroxides such as hydrogen peroxide, which can also exert powerful chemical effects on biological tissues.

ROS are involved in many beneficial and essential processes in the body, including our immune response. But they can also cause damage on the cellular level when they occur persistently enough or in large enough numbers to overwhelm the body's natural defense system of antioxidants—the various enzymes and small molecules that are designed to bond with and neutralize ROS. These built-in defenses have developed naturally, reflecting the fact we live in an oxygen-rich environment and use oxygen as a primary source in our metabolic activities. The damage caused by overabundant ROS is called oxidative stress, and it is thought to play an important role in the aging process. In addition, oxidative stress has been linked to cancer, neurodegenerative diseases, inflammatory conditions such as arthritis, and atherosclerosis, which is a major cause of cardiovascular disease.

Oxidative stress also appears to contribute to the blood vessel damage and other complications caused by elevated blood glucose levels in someone with poorly controlled type 1 or type 2 diabetes. Because of their role in diabetic complications, the scientists at Joslin have spent many years investigating how the effects of ROS can be controlled and prevented. More recently, researchers have uncovered evidence that ROS may also be contributing to insulin resistance and pancreatic damage associated with the onset of type 1 and 2 diabetes. One of the most

The Importance of Vitamin D

Although it's not technically an antioxidant, having a sufficient level of vitamin D is important for your overall health, including the strength of your immune system, and for your glucose metabolism. In one recent meta-analysis of twenty-one studies involving more than 76,000 individuals, the investigators found a significant inverse association between blood levels of vitamin D and diabetes risk. Low vitamin D levels have also been linked to increased risk for metabolic syndrome and impaired fasting glucose.

Interestingly, studies now suggest that a majority of people who live in northern latitudes have low levels of vitamin D for much of the year, most likely because they're not being exposed to enough sunlight to stimulate their body's natural vitamin D production—a fact that may be related to the increased risk at these latitudes that has been observed for certain conditions such as prostate cancer, multiple sclerosis, and irritable bowel syndrome. For this reason, I recommend having your vitamin D levels checked by your doctor and taking a prescription supplement if your levels are low.

important recent discoveries regarding these mechanisms, in fact, was also made by Dr. Kahn, along with his Joslin research team.

At the same time, as mentioned earlier, ROS perform many important beneficial tasks as well. This fact explains why studies have found that taking a large daily dose of one or two isolated antioxidants such as vitamin C or vitamin E is highly problematic and can often cause as much harm as good. It also explains why many diabetes researchers are now focusing instead on how to trigger the activity of the body's own natural antioxidants, which include many specialized types of molecules that work on the cellular level in sophisticated ways.

What the Research Shows

A number of large-scale studies have found that people who eat more antioxidant-rich foods or have higher levels of antioxidants in their bodies appear to be at decreased risk for developing type 2 diabetes. At the same time, researchers are linking ROS activity to a wide range of processes associated with the development of insulin resistance.

PEOPLE WITH HIGHER LEVELS OF ANTIOXIDANTS ARE LESS LIKELY TO DEVELOP METABOLIC SYNDROME.

In 2011, investigators at the NIH's National Institute for Aging published an analysis of NHANES data from 2001 to 2006, based on detailed examinations of nearly twelve thousand Americans. They found that men and women with the highest blood levels of carotenoids and vitamin C, compounds that are potent antioxidants, were least likely to have metabolic syndrome—a cluster of conditions associated with significantly increased risk for developing type 2 diabetes. The researchers also found that those in the survey who were diagnosed with metabolic syndrome tended to have low blood levels of vitamin D and elevated levels of the amino acid homocysteine—both of which are a sign of increased oxidative stress. The same researchers later published an analysis of nearly eight hundred American adolescents ages twelve to nineteen and found a link between increased levels of carotenoids and vitamin C and reduced risk for metabolic syndrome.

PEOPLE WHO EAT DIETS HIGH IN ANTIOXIDANTS ARE LESS LIKELY TO HAVE SIGNS OF INSULIN RESISTANCE AND IMPAIRED GLUCOSE CONTROL.

In another recently published study, Greek researchers looked at a subset of more than one thousand men and women from the well-known ATTICA Study. They found that eating a diet higher in antioxidant-rich foods correlated with better glucose control and insulin sensitivity, including lower blood levels of glucose and insulin as well as reduced markers of insulin resistance.

OXIDATIVE STRESS APPEARS TO HAVE A KEY ROLE IN INSULIN RESISTANCE CAUSED BY INFLAMMATION AND STRESS HORMONES.

In a 2006 paper published in the journal *Nature,* investigators at MIT and Harvard induced insulin resistance in lab mice in two different ways—by administering the cytokine TNF-α (mimicking the insulin resistant–causing effects of inflammation) to one group and by treating the other group with the glucocorticoid dexamethasone (which has a biochemical effect similar to that of cortisol, the stress hormone greatly elevated in people experiencing chronic stress). They then analyzed the genomes of the two animal models and found that ROS levels were increased in both of them. Next, the researchers took a group of mice that had been bred for obesity and insulin resistance and administered a drug treatment designed to reduce ROS activity. They found that the treatment improved insulin sensitivity and glucose control in the mice. Other studies have confirmed that insulin resistance caused by the inflammatory cytokine TNF-α appears to be mediated by oxidative stress and by the ROS hydrogen peroxide in particular.

OXIDATIVE STRESS MAY BE THE KEY LINK BETWEEN A HIGH-FAT DIET AND INSULIN RESISTANCE.

Japanese researchers have demonstrated that when insulin resistance is induced in laboratory mice by feeding them a high-fat diet, this stimulates their genes to begin generating more ROS and more oxidative stress in their fat and liver cells *before* insulin resistance actually sets in.

OXIDATIVE STRESS MAY BE A CAUSE OF INSULIN RESISTANCE IN THE SKELETAL MUSCLES.

Investigators in France have found fascinating evidence that impaired mitochondrial function in the skeletal muscles—which, as we've seen, is one of the factors linked to insulin resistance in the muscles—may actually be a result rather than a cause of insulin resistance and that these impairments may actually be due to oxidative stress produced by the prediabetic state. When the researchers fed lab mice a high-fat, high-sugar diet, the mice first developed insulin resistance and then prediabetes and type 2 diabetes, as expected. The defects in the mice's mitochondria, however, did not appear until their prediabetes had actually progressed to full-blown diabetes. The researchers also found that this mitochondrial dysfunction was preceded by ROS production and oxidative stress in the muscles of the lab animals and that when they blocked this ROS production with antioxidants, the mitochondrial defects did not occur.

OXIDATIVE STRESS APPEARS TO BE A FACTOR IN THE INSULIN RESISTANCE CAUSED BY NONALCOHOLIC FATTY LIVER DISEASE.

As noted in Strategy Chapter 2, the buildup of fat deposits in the liver appears to be both a cause and a result of insulin resistance, creating a vicious cycle that helps spur the progression of type 2 diabetes in people with impaired glucose metabolism. In a reflection of this link, nonalcoholic fatty liver disease has been increasing at epidemic rates, in parallel with the type 2 diabetes epidemic. Study of the signaling cascade involved in fatty liver has concluded that oxidative stress plays a key role in promoting the inflammation and insulin resistance associated with this condition. This finding carries special importance because there is currently no effective medication for nonalcoholic fatty liver. If oxidative stress is a major factor in its development, then treatment with antioxidants could be an option.

The bottom line: ROS appear to play a contributing role in causing insulin resistance, and they do so through a variety of different mechanisms.

Oxidative Stress and Diabetic Complications

I n addition to its role in causing type 2 diabetes, oxidative stress has also been clearly implicated as a major source of the damage caused to the blood vessels and other organs by elevated blood glucose levels. It's now believed that increased production of ROS in the mitochondria due to hyperglycemia plays a major role in this process. In addition, elevated glucose levels can activate a series of enzymes that stimulate production of ROS, further contributing to blood vessel and organ damage.

The bottom line: ROS produced by elevated blood glucose levels play an important role in the tissue damage associated with diabetes-related complications.

How to Increase Your Own Natural Antioxidant Production with "Phase 2 Antioxidants"

A ll of these intriguing discoveries about how oxidative stress contributes to impaired glucose metabolism have naturally led scientists to examine whether treating people with antioxidants can help improve their insulin sensitivity and prevent them from developing type 2 diabetes. Although off-the-shelf antioxidants appear to work against ROS-induced insulin resistance in the lab, however, the results of human trials have been less promising. (See box on page 204: The Limited Benefits of Vitamins E and C.)

Given the wide variety of ROS in the body, it makes intuitive sense that simply picking individual antioxidants and setting them loose in the body will have limited effect. In addition, oxidative stress tends to take place on the cellular level and involves mind-boggling numbers of ROS. Swallowing an antioxidant supplement and hoping that enough of that compound will consistently make it through the digestive system and the bloodstream to the site of all this oxidative activity is something of a long shot, to say the least. In fact, a number of important natural antioxidants can't survive being digested and are available only when they're produced naturally in the body.

What *does* have scientists excited, on the other hand, is the concept of inducing your body to ramp up production of its own army of antioxidants. Not only are these natural antioxidants both numerous and widely diverse, but they are also manufactured and act on the cellular level, where they are most needed.

The key to this approach involves substances called Phase 2 antioxidants. These compounds don't exert a direct antioxidant action themselves, but instead boost activity of the body's own antioxidant defenses. They work by activating a protein called nrf2 (its full name is a jawbreaker: *nuclear factor erythroid 2–related factor 2*). Discovered in 2002 by Johns Hopkins researchers, nrf2 is what's known as a transcription factor, meaning that it acts as a powerful "genetic switch," working in the nucleus of the cell to turn on (express) different sets of genes in your cells that are responsible for manufacturing a wide array of natural antioxidants. If you think of oxidative stress as being like a billion tiny fires inside your cells, the effect is like sending an automatic signal that makes billions of sprinklers go off inside each burning room, instead of having the fire department spray water against the building's outside wall.

Nrf2 also activates genes with anti-inflammatory properties, which is why Phase 2 antioxidants also tend to be effective at helping to reduce inflammation—another key strategy for reversing insulin resistance and type 2 diabetes, as outlined in Strategy Chapter 5.

Phase 2 antioxidants are actually types of phytonutrients—the thousands of healing compounds contained in plants. By the way, the sheer variety of these phytonutrients helps explain why a diet

Nrf2 Activator Supplements

A couple of nrf2 activator supplements are commercially available, each of which contains a mixture of several phytonutrients that are known to stimulate nrf2 activity:

- *Nrf2 Activator*, manufactured by the company Health Naturally, contains sulforaphane, curcumin, pterostilbene, and green tea extract.

- *Protandim*, manufactured by the company LiveVantage, contains ashgawanda root, bacopa extract, milk thistle extract, green tea extract, and turmeric extract.

of healthy foods will provide more benefits than any single supplement ever could—which is one of the reasons why the RAD eating plan, which stresses foods rich in phytonutrients, is so good for your health. These phytonutrients also appear to have a synergistic effect, meaning that you'll get more benefits from eating a number of these foods in combination, and their nrf2-boosting benefits can last up to twenty-four hours.

Following is a list of foods that are particularly good sources of Phase 2 antioxidants:

BROCCOLI, BRUSSELS SPROUTS, CAULIFLOWER, AND CABBAGE

All cruciferous vegetables, including broccoli, Brussels sprouts, cauliflower, and cabbage, contain large quantities of sulforaphane, a potent Phase 2 antioxidant and the most widely studied of all nrf2 activators. Of these vegetables, broccoli is the sulforaphane champion, and its dark green florettes are where most of that sulforaphane is found. *Broccoli sprouts* offer an even more concentrated source of sulforaphane and are commonly used as a source of sulforaphane in research projects. Another concentrated source is *broccoli seed extract,* which can be purchased from health food stores.

Seven "Antidiabetes" Supplements That Are More Hype Than Help

Magazine articles and the Internet are filled with advice about various nutritional supplements that can supposedly help people with type 2 diabetes achieve better blood glucose control. Most of these claims have no real evidence behind them, however, and the supplements themselves are a waste of money at best. The following nutritional supplements have all been touted for their ability to improve glucose metabolism—yet there's no proof that any of them have any actual benefits:

- Chromium
- Magnesium
- Vanadium
- CoQ10
- Alpha Lipoic acid
- Vitamin K
- Resveratrol

BLUEBERRIES

They contain large amounts of the phytonutrient pterostilbene, which is a very effective nrf2 activator.

SALMON, TUNA, SARDINES, MACKEREL, AND HERRING

All of these fatty fish contain the omega-3 fatty acids DHA (docosahexae-noic acid) and EPA (eicosapentaenoic acid), both of which significantly boost nrf2 activity. You can also obtain DHA and EPA in concentrated form in *fish oil, krill oil, algal oil,* and *flaxseed oil.* Besides their antioxi-dant-promoting benefits, DHA and EPA have potent anti-inflammatory properties as well.

GREEN TEA

Green tea contains a wide array of antioxidants in its own right and also stimulates the nrf2 pathway. For a more concentrated dose of its active ingredients you can take a supplement containing *green tea extract,* widely available in health food stores.

CURCUMIN

This nutrient, the active ingredient of the Indian spice turmeric, has a powerful stimulating effect on the nrft2 pathway. (As noted in Strategy Chapter 5, it is a powerful inflammation-fighting food as well.) *Turmeric extract* will also provide a concentrated source of this phytonutrient.

COFFEE

A number of studies have found that various types of coffee beans have the potential to activate the nrf2 pathway. This effect appears to vary according to how the coffee beans are roasted, however, with dark roasted coffee showing significantly more beneficial activity. The effect also appears to differ somewhat from person to person. Given Americans' propensity for their morning cup of java, we can expect to see a good deal more research in this area.

STRAWBERRIES

Researchers in Britain report that they were able to show that *strawberry extract* activates the nrf2 pathway. Obviously, that means straight-up strawberries do the trick as well.

HERBAL SUPPLEMENTS

As additional sources of Phase 2 antioxidants, you can also take supplements of *silymarin* (contained in the herb *milk thistle*), as well as the Ayurvedic herbs *bacopa extract* and *ashwagandha root powder,* which can be readily found in health food stores or purchased online.

Harnessing the Healing Power of Plants

A lthough I recommend making a special effort to eat plenty of these nrf2-activating foods for the reasons explained in this chapter, I don't want to downplay the many other phytonutrients in plants—all of which have antioxidant, anti-inflammatory, and antiviral properties that will enable you to maintain optimal health. The Rural Asian Diet outlined in Strategy Chapter 1 is designed to help you incorporate a wide range of these plants into your daily menu. Any single fruit, vegetable, or grain contains thousands of these nutrients, offering a nutritional banquet that no pill or supplement can match. The best approach is to eat a large variety of unprocessed plant foods in all the colors of the rainbow. By following this plan, you will be laying the strongest possible foundation for a long, healthy, active, and energy-filled life.

Oxidative Stress and Brain Health

P hase 2 antioxidants are also important for maintaining brain health because the brain accounts for 20% of the body's oxygen consumption, making it especially vulnerable to oxidative stress. In fact, damage from ROS has now been implicated in virtually every degenerative brain condition, including Alzheimer's, amyotrophic lateral sclerosis (ALS, or Lou Gehrig's disease), and Parkinson's disease. This connection is particularly important for people with type 2 diabetes because they are at heightened risk of developing Alzheimer's disease, for reasons that remain unclear. (Although it is controversial, high doses of vitamin E have also been reported to delay the progression of Alzheimer's.)

PART 2

PUTTING THE DIABETES RESET STRATEGIES INTO ACTION:
A Twelve-Week Implementation Plan

Prediabetes and Type 2 Diabetes: Multiple Causes Require a Mix of Strategies

In Part One of *The Diabetes Reset,* I discussed the many different factors that can affect your glucose metabolism, along with the various measures you can take to neutralize these factors. One of the goals of this book is to help you understand that type 2 diabetes and its precursor, prediabetes, have multiple causes that work in combination, first to gradually reduce your insulin sensitivity, and then eventually to diminish the ability of your pancreas to produce insulin as well. The exact mix of factors is different for everyone. What is causing your prediabetes or type 2 diabetes is determined in part by which risk factors you have and in part by how genetically vulnerable you are to these risk factors.

Because insulin resistance, prediabetes, and diabetes are caused by multiple factors, I encourage anyone who is concerned about their glucose metabolism to employ as many of the strategies in this book as they can. Every one of these strategies, pursued on its own, is likely to lower your diabetes risk, and each strategy is also good for your health in other ways. Pursue them all together and you're significantly more likely to achieve excellent general health and diminished risk of diabetes.

Having said that, it also makes sense to focus most closely on the strategies that will benefit your own individual situation the most. To some extent, you can find out which of these strategies will work best for you only by actually implementing them. The following quiz, however, can help you pinpoint which risk factors are most likely to be affecting your body's ability to process glucose.

Diabetes Reset Target Strategy Quiz: What Should You Be Focusing On?

G ive yourself 4 points for every (a) answer, 3 points for every (b), 2 points for every (c), and 1 point for every (d).

A. DIET

1. **How many fiber-rich foods (whole grains, vegetables, legumes, and fruit) do you eat each day?**

   a. I eat practically no fiber-rich foods.

   b. I eat a small amount of fiber most days.

   c. I eat some fiber at every meal.

   d. I eat a considerable amount of fiber at every meal.

2. **How much refined carbohydrates (white bread, white rice, sugar-flavored drinks and snacks, non-whole-grain pasta, commercial baked goods) do you eat each day?**

   a. I eat a considerable amount of these foods at every meal.

   b. I eat some of these foods at every meal.

   c. I eat a small amount of these foods most days.

   d. I hardly ever eat these foods.

3. **How much non-heart healthy fat (non-low-fat cheese, milk, and ice cream, eggs with yolks, butter, chicken with skin, steak, ground beef, hot dogs, bacon, sausage, commercial baked goods, potato chips, fried foods) do you eat?**

   a. I eat a considerable amount of these foods at every meal.

   b. I eat some of these foods at every meal.

   c. I eat a small amount of these foods most days.

   d. I hardly ever eat these foods.

8 TO 12 POINTS: You are eating too much fat and too little fiber. Shifting to the RAD eating plan's high-fiber, low-fat diet by following the Diabetes Reset Healthy Eating Track should be a top priority.

5 TO 8 POINTS: Your eating pattern is fairly healthy, but there is still room to increase your fiber intake and cut down on dietary fat by implementing the RAD eating plan via the Diabetes Reset Healthy Eating Track.

4 POINTS: You are already following a healthy dietary strategy. Use the RAD eating plan as an ongoing guide to make sure you continue optimizing your fiber intake while holding your fat consumption down to the safest level possible.

B. BODY WEIGHT

1. **Based on the chart on page 72, my BMI is:**

   a. 35 or above

   b. Between 30 and 35

   c. Between 25 and 30

   d. Below 25

2. **I would describe my shape as:**

   a. Very apple shaped (I have a large, round belly and midsection.)

   b. Somewhat apple shaped

   c. Pear shaped (I have excess fat in my thighs and buttocks but not my midsection.)

   d. Slim (neither apple nor pear shaped)

3. **Which describes your condition?**

   a. I've been diagnosed with type 2 diabetes.

   b. I have prediabetes.

c. My insulin levels are elevated, indicating that I have insulin resistance, but my glucose levels are in normal range.

d. I have normal blood levels of insulin and glucose.

7 TO 12 POINTS: You are overweight, and it is affecting your blood glucose control. I strongly recommend following the Diabetes Reset Weight-Loss Track as well as the Healthy Eating Track.

5 TO 7 POINTS: Although following the Diabetes Reset Weight-Loss Track isn't essential, you could benefit from reducing your weight somewhat.

4 POINTS: You don't need to utilize the Diabetes Reset Weight-Loss Track at this time.

C. EXERCISE

1. **During my normal daily activities, I would describe myself as:**

   a. Not active at all—I do almost no walking during the day.

   b. Occasionally active—I walk some, but no more than is absolutely necessary.

   c. Somewhat active—I spend a fair amount of each day on my feet and walking.

   d. Very active—I'm always standing and walking about.

2. **How many hours do you spend sitting each day?**

   a. Ten hours or more

   b. Five to ten hours, with occasional breaks to stand up and walk about

   c. Five to ten hours, with frequent standing and walking breaks

   d. Less than five hours

3. **How often do you do a planned session of aerobic exercise?**

   a. I never do aerobic exercise.

   b. I do some aerobic exercise one to three days each week.

c. I do some aerobic exercise four to six days per week.

d. I do at least twenty-five minutes of aerobic exercise four to six days per week.

10 TO 12 POINTS: You are doing far too little exercise and can significantly improve your health through a program of daily physical activity. I recommend starting the Diabetes Reset Aerobic Exercise Track at Week 1 and starting the Strength Training Track when you feel ready for it.

6 TO 9 POINTS: You are already getting in some daily physical activity, which is good. I recommend starting the Diabetes Reset Aerobic Exercise Track at Week 2 and starting the Strength Training Track in Week 4 as scheduled.

4 TO 5 POINTS: You currently have a healthy level of physical activity. To continue and perhaps increase your activity level and ensure that you're getting enough exercise to optimize your glucose metabolism, I recommend starting the Diabetes Reset Aerobic Exercise Track at Week 3 and starting the Strength Training Track in Week 4 as scheduled.

D. INFLAMMATION

1. My gums are:

    a. Very red and tender, and always bleed when I brush them

    b. Somewhat red and tender and bleed occasionally

    c. Slightly red and tender

    d. Normal

2. Have you been diagnosed with asthma or an inflammatory autoimmune disorder such as rheumatoid arthritis, psoriasis, or inflammatory bowel disease—and if so, how would you describe it?

    a. Yes, and it is persistent with severe symptoms.

    b. Yes, and it is persistent but with mild symptoms.

    c. Yes, but I have only occasional mild symptoms.

    d. No, I have not been diagnosed with any of these conditions.

3. **How often do you suffer from infections?**

    a. Constantly

    b. Occasionally

    c. Rarely

    d. Almost never

8 TO 12 POINTS: You most likely have some degree of chronic inflammation. The Diabetes Reset Inflammation-Fighting Track should be a top priority.

5 TO 7 POINTS: You may have a low level of chronic inflammation and will definitely benefit from following the Diabetes Reset Inflammation-Fighting Track.

4 POINTS: Chronic inflammation is most likely not an issue, although your general health could still benefit from the tips outlined in the Diabetes Reset Inflammation-Fighting Track.

E. SLEEP

1. **How would you describe your typical night's sleep?**

    a. I get six hours of sleep or less and often wake up feeling tired.

    b. I get at least seven hours of sleep but often wake up feeling less than rested.

    c. I get six hours or less of sleep but usually wake up feeling rested.

    d. I get at least seven hours of sleep and usually wake up feeling rested.

2. **Have you been told you snore, and if so, how is your snoring described?**

   a. I snore severely and frequently.

   b. I occasionally snore severely.

   c. I occasionally snore, but not severely.

   d. I never snore.

3. **Which of these describes how you typically feel during the day?**

   a. I feel sleepy much of the time.

   b. I feel sleepy some of the time.

   c. I feel sleepy once in a while.

   d. I always feel alert and well rested.

8 TO 12 POINTS: Your sleep quality and amount is not good, and you may well be suffering from sleep apnea. The Diabetes Reset Healthy Sleep Track should be a top priority.

5 TO 7 POINTS: Your sleep quality and amount could be improved. I strongly recommend following the Diabetes Reset Healthy Sleep Track.

4 TO 5 POINTS: Your sleep quality is good and you are getting a healthy amount of sleep. You don't need to utilize the Diabetes Reset Healthy Sleep Track at this time.

F. STRESS

1. **How would you rate your daily stress level, including work, home life, and other responsibilities?**

   a. High

   b. Moderate

   c. Generally low with occasional moments of higher stress

   d. Almost always low

2. **How would you rate your job in terms of stress?**

   a. Very stressful

   b. Somewhat stressful

   c. A little bit stressful

   d. Not stressful at all

3. **Have you experienced a very stressful event in your life over the past five years, such as the death of a loved one, loss of a job, divorce, or a financial setback?**

   a. Yes, I've experienced more than one such event.

   b. Yes, I've experienced one such event.

   c. Yes, I've experienced one such event, but it was several years ago and I'm over it now.

   d. No, I've not experienced such an event.

8 TO 12 POINTS: You are at risk of health damage from chronic stress. The Diabetes Reset Anti-Stress Track should be a top priority.

5 TO 7 POINTS: You could benefit from stress reduction techniques. I strongly recommend following the Diabetes Reset Anti-Stress Track.

4 POINTS: Stress doesn't appear to be an issue. You probably don't need to utilize the Diabetes Reset Healthy Sleep Track at this time, although you may find that your mood and health will benefit from some stress-reduction techniques anyway.

A Twelve-Week Plan for Improving Your Glucose Metabolism

This twelve-week Diabetes Reset Plan is designed for someone who is overweight, eating a high-fat, low-fiber diet, and doing almost no exercise of any kind—who, in short, is starting from square one. It includes a number of different tracks, each one based on a different strategy for enhancing your organs' insulin sensitivity and protecting your insulin-producing beta cells. The tracks are:

The Twelve-Week Diabetes Reset Plan at a Glance

The Diabetes Reset Plan starts with major lifestyle strategies such as diet, exercise, and weight loss, then introduces other strategies gradually over the course of the twelve weeks:

TRACK/START WEEK	1	2	3	4	5	6	7	8	9	10	11	12
Healthy Eating	•	•	•	•	•	•	•	•	•	•	•	•
Weight Loss	•	•	•	•	•	•	•	•	•	•	•	•
Aerobic Exercise Level I	•	•	•	•	•	•	•	•	•	•	•	•
Aerobic Exercise Level II							•	•	•	•	•	•
Strength Training				•	•	•	•	•	•	•	•	•
Inflammation Fighting					•	•	•	•	•	•	•	•
Healthy Sleep						•	•	•	•	•	•	•
Anti-Stress								•	•	•	•	•
Natural Antioxidants									•	•	•	•
Brown Fat Activation										•	•	•
Vitamin D											•	•

- A **Healthy Eating Track**, to help you begin shifting your daily eating patterns toward the Rural Asian Diet model of low-fat, high-fiber meals and snacks

- A **Weight-Loss Track**, for readers who want to reduce their body weight

- An **Aerobic Exercise Track** and a **Strength Training Track** that will show you how to increase your physical activity level in a safe and gradual fashion

- An **Inflammation-Fighting Track** that focuses on identifying and treating any sources of inflammation in your body

- A **Healthy Sleep Track** to help you address any sleep problems you may be having

- An **Anti-Stress Track** that will help you incorporate stress-reducing strategies into your daily routine

- A **Natural Antioxidants Track** to keep your body's natural defenses strong

- A **Brown Fat Activation Track** to maximize your brown fat's calorie-burning potential

- A **Vitamin D Track** for anyone who is deficient in this key nutrient

How to Use the Diabetes Reset Weekly Calendars

Each weekly guide for the Diabetes Reset Plan includes a calendar to track your progress. You can use this calendar to note your daily physical activity totals, daily grams of dietary fiber, fat and total calories, and other notations about your progress, including hours slept and blood glucose levels, if you're measuring them. The pages are also available for download at workman.com/thediabetesreset.

Week 1: Time to Get Moving!

GOALS FOR THE WEEK

- Take an inventory of your eating patterns and begin reducing your fat intake while increasing your dietary fiber to 20 grams per day.

- Begin to develop your daily "intentional walking" routine, starting this week at 1,500 steps/fifteen minutes per day for six days out of the week, with one rest day.

Week 1: Overview

HEALTHY EATING TRACK

DIAL UP THE FIBER, DIAL DOWN THE FAT. That is the essential Diabetes Reset nutritional message for this week, this year, and the rest of your life. If you can start eating at least 30 grams of fiber each day, while keeping your fat intake close to 15% of your total calories, I guarantee you will see a swift and lasting improvement in your blood glucose control. My only caution is to increase your fiber intake to that level over a couple of weeks and drink plenty of water while doing so, if you aren't there already. This will give your digestive system time to adjust to added fiber while avoiding potential side effects like bloating, gas, or intestinal discomfort.

It's also a good idea to start by taking stock of your current eating pattern: For the first three days of this week, I want you to eat as you normally do and keep a record of everything you consume in the Daily Eating Record that accompanies this week's calendar (see page 230). Keep track in the notepad section of your smartphone or in a notebook, or download the form located at workman.com/thediabetesreset: Write down the type and amount of every item of food and drink you consume on these days.

When you've finished your record for each day, go to the RAD food list that starts on page 56, and calculate the total grams of fiber contained in the vegetables, fruits, legumes, and grain products that you ate during the day. Write this amount on your daily food record. Next, identify the high-fat foods, including any non-low-fat dairy products, egg yolks, chicken with the skin intact, fried foods, commercial baked goods, processed meats, or snack foods such as chips that you ate during the day. You can use the high-fat foods listed in Tip 1 on the next page as a starting point.

After you've completed your daily food record for three days, take a few minutes to study how many vegetables, legumes, whole grains, and fruits you're consuming at each meal, and also what your main sources of dietary fat are.

NEXT: BEGIN YOUR SHIFT TO EATING LESS FAT AND MORE FIBER. For the last four days of the week, look for every opportunity you can to consume less fat at each meal and snack, using the suggestions in Strategy Chapter 1 and the tips that follow. At the same time, begin heading toward your ultimate fiber intake goal by aiming to eat 20 grams of fiber in each of these four days, using the RAD food list as your guide. Record the estimated total grams of fat and fiber that you eat each day in your weekly record.

GLUCOSE CHECK 1

During this four-day period, I recommend picking two days and using a blood glucose home test kit to check your blood glucose levels four times each day—when you first wake up, and then again one hour after each meal. Write down these two sets of readings along with the average of the two sets, and file them away in your computer or smartphone. They will serve as a baseline to help you gauge how your Diabetes Reset strategies are working over the next twelve weeks.

TIPS FOR THE WEEK: *Beware the fat traps.* Begin making a habit of avoiding especially high-fat foods: bacon, potato chips, cheddar cheese, corned beef, ground beef, bologna, chicken with the skin on, high-fat ice cream, beef hot dogs, croissants, doughnuts, high-fat mayonnaise, butter, steak, high-fat cream cheese.

Practice fat substitution. To help keep your fat intake low, start incorporating these low-fat substitutes into your daily diet: skim milk, low-fat cheeses, yogurt, and ice cream, light mayonnaise, low-sodium soy sauce and teriyaki sauce (instead of cooking oils), egg whites without the yolks or egg substitute, fat-free butter substitutes.

WEIGHT-LOSS TRACK

If you're planning to follow the Diabetes Reset Weight-Loss Track, for now simply follow the Healthy Eating Track as you begin shifting to a lower-fat, higher-fiber eating pattern. In Week 3, the Weight-Loss Track will break away from the Healthy Eating Track by adding a calorie-restriction element. It's a good idea, however, to start noticing your portion sizes. See page 95 for a list of the sizes of standard portions.

AEROBIC EXERCISE TRACK LEVEL I

If you haven't been engaging in any regular physical activity for some time, you first need to get clearance from your regular doctor to begin an exercise program. Once you have that green light, your second move should be to buy a good pair of walking shoes. Your goal this week is to begin your progress toward Level I of aerobic activity (150 minutes per week of moderate-intensity aerobic exercise) by walking 1,500 "intentional" steps on six out of every seven days. This is equivalent to fifteen minutes of walking at a brisk pace per day. Note that this walking is *in addition to* the five thousand or so daily "incidental" steps (the more casual walking you do in the course of normal life) that the average person routinely puts in. You can fit in your fifteen minutes of brisk walking any way you like—even in segments as short as a few minutes. Your effort during these segments should be moderately intense—a 10 to 13 on the Perceived Exertion scale (see page 120) but never so hard that you can't easily carry on a conversation as you walk.

At the same time, I encourage you to make sure you're getting your full five thousand steps of incidental walking each day as well. In particular, be sure to break up any long stretches of sitting with at least a minute or two of walking. If you haven't already, this would be an excellent time to purchase a pedometer to track both your intentional and incidental walking (see page 119).

TIP FOR THE WEEK: *Don't overdo it.* As noted previously, aerobic exercise is meant to be enjoyable, despite what you hear from the exercise gurus espousing "Marine boot camp"–type workouts. The Diabetes Reset Plan calls for maintaining a moderate, conversational pace, one that will raise your heartbeat to a pleasant rate of 100 to 130 beats per minute and have you sweating slightly. If your workout starts to feel too hard, simply ease up on the pace a bit.

Daily Eating Record

DAY 1

Total grams of fiber _____   High-fat foods _____

BREAKFAST	SNACK	LUNCH	SNACK	DINNER	SNACK

DAY 2

Total grams of fiber _____   High-fat foods _____

BREAKFAST	SNACK	LUNCH	SNACK	DINNER	SNACK

DAY 3

Total grams of fiber _____   High-fat foods _____

BREAKFAST	SNACK	LUNCH	SNACK	DINNER	SNACK

Diabetes Reset Calendar—Week 1

DAY 1

DAILY AEROBIC ACTIVITY

My walking windows

Minutes _____   Steps _____

Minutes _____   Steps _____

Minutes _____   Steps _____

Minutes _____   Steps _____

Minutes _____   Steps _____

Total grams of fiber eaten _____

High-fat foods eaten _____

DAY 2

DAILY AEROBIC ACTIVITY

My walking windows

Minutes _____   Steps _____

Minutes _____   Steps _____

Minutes _____   Steps _____

Minutes _____   Steps _____

Minutes _____   Steps _____

Total grams of fiber eaten _____

High-fat foods eaten _____

DAY 3

DAILY AEROBIC ACTIVITY

My walking windows

Minutes _____   Steps _____

Minutes _____   Steps _____

Minutes _____   Steps _____

Minutes _____   Steps _____

Minutes _____   Steps _____

Total grams of fiber eaten _____

High-fat foods eaten _____

DAY 4

DAILY AEROBIC ACTIVITY

My walking windows

Minutes _____   Steps _____

Minutes _____   Steps _____

Minutes _____   Steps _____

Minutes _____   Steps _____

Minutes _____   Steps _____

Total grams of fiber eaten _____

High-fat foods eaten _____

DAY 5

DAILY AEROBIC ACTIVITY

My walking windows

Minutes _____   Steps _____

Minutes _____   Steps _____

Minutes _____   Steps _____

Minutes _____   Steps _____

Minutes _____   Steps _____

Total grams of fiber eaten _____

High-fat foods eaten _____

DAY 6

DAILY AEROBIC ACTIVITY

My walking windows

Minutes _____   Steps _____

Minutes _____   Steps _____

Minutes _____   Steps _____

Minutes _____   Steps _____

Minutes _____   Steps _____

Total grams of fiber eaten _____

High-fat foods eaten _____

DAY 7

DAILY AEROBIC ACTIVITY

My walking windows

Minutes _____   Steps _____

Minutes _____   Steps _____

Minutes _____   Steps _____

Minutes _____   Steps _____

Minutes _____   Steps _____

Total grams of fiber eaten _____

High-fat foods eaten _____

Week 2: Kicking Off Your RAD Eating Plan

GOALS FOR THE WEEK

- Continue implementing the Rural Asian Diet, increasing your daily fiber intake to 25 grams per day as you begin to employ the RAD meal plans outlined in Part One of *The Diabetes Reset*.

- Increase your daily amount of intentional walking by five hundred steps/five minutes, so that you are walking two thousand steps/twenty minutes per day for six days this week, with one rest day.

Week 2: Overview

HEALTHY EATING TRACK

You're off to a great start! In Week 2, you'll continue looking for ways to reduce the amount of fat and increase the amount of fiber you eat each day. This week, ramp up your daily fiber intake slightly each day until you're consuming 25 grams of fiber per day at week's end, as you continue to focus on eating more whole grains, non-starchy vegetables, and legumes. Begin the week by using the RAD meal plans list, which begins on page 63, to plan your meals and snacks for the week, then make a trip to your local market to shop for the ingredients in your menu plan.

TIP FOR THE WEEK: *Make high-fiber foods a centerpiece of every meal.* Not only is dietary fiber itself good for you, but foods high in fiber are also rich in many other vital nutrients. Try to incorporate as much fiber into each meal as possible, starting with these high-fiber favorites: green beans, lima beans, fava beans, kidney beans, black beans, lentils, baked beans, chickpeas, hummus, broccoli, sweet potatoes, winter squash, spinach, collard greens, parsnips, peas, high-fiber bran cereals and bran muffins, cooked whole grains, whole-grain bread and pasta, bran muffins, raspberries, blueberries, bananas, oranges, or apples (with the skin).

WEIGHT-LOSS TRACK

If you're planning to follow the Diabetes Reset Weight-Loss Track, continue following the Healthy Eating Track for now. Next week, the Weight-Loss Track will add a calorie-restriction element to your eating plan.

AEROBIC EXERCISE TRACK LEVEL I

By increasing your fiber consumption, decreasing your fat intake, and becoming more physically active every day, you have already begun to reset the way your body processes glucose. This week, your exercise prescription is to keep your momentum going by adding another five hundred steps/five minutes to your daily total of intentional walking, so that you're doing two thousand steps or twenty minutes of steady, brisk walking each day. This second week of physical activity is a time to pay special attention to your body. If you have any aches or pains, that's a sign to take an extra day off from your walking program. Either take a rest day or switch to a low-impact form of exercise such as riding a bicycle or stationary bike or swimming for twenty minutes. If the pain persists, see a doctor.

TIP FOR THE WEEK: *Dress for success.* Your daily exercise session should be a pleasant experience—never an ordeal. Dressing for comfort and mobility will help ensure that this is the case. In addition to well-fitted, well-constructed workout shoes, develop an exercise wardrobe of comfortable short- and long-sleeved T-shirts, shorts and a comfortable pair of loose-fitting trousers or sweat pants, and a sweatshirt or warm-up jacket for cool weather. Add a baseball cap or sunglasses on extremely sunny days, a rain suit to walk outside in rainy weather, and a knit cap and gloves in cold winter months. For extra protection against the cold, buy long underwear tops and bottoms made with polypropylene—a synthetic fiber that has remarkable wicking properties, meaning that it directs sweat away from your skin surface, leaving it dry and toasty. (For especially cold days, consider heading to a nearby mall or other indoor area suitable for extended walking.)

Diabetes Reset Calendar—Week 2

DAY 1

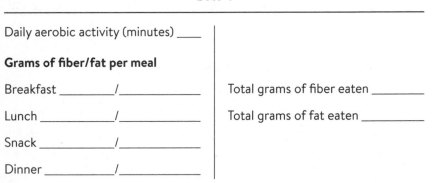

Daily aerobic activity (minutes) _____

Grams of fiber/fat per meal

Breakfast _____ / _____   Total grams of fiber eaten _____

Lunch _____ / _____   Total grams of fat eaten _____

Snack _____ / _____

Dinner _____ / _____

DAY 2

Daily aerobic activity (minutes) _____

Grams of fiber/fat per meal

Breakfast _____/_____   Total grams of fiber eaten _____

Lunch _____/_____   Total grams of fat eaten _____

Snack _____/_____

Dinner _____/_____

DAY 3

Daily aerobic activity (minutes) _____

Grams of fiber/fat per meal

Breakfast _____/_____   Total grams of fiber eaten _____

Lunch _____/_____   Total grams of fat eaten _____

Snack _____/_____

Dinner _____/_____

DAY 4

Daily aerobic activity (minutes) _____

Grams of fiber/fat per meal

Breakfast _____/_____   Total grams of fiber eaten _____

Lunch _____/_____   Total grams of fat eaten _____

Snack _____/_____

Dinner _____/_____

DAY 5

Daily aerobic activity (minutes) _____

Grams of fiber/fat per meal

Breakfast _____/_____   Total grams of fiber eaten _____

Lunch _____/_____   Total grams of fat eaten _____

Snack _____/_____

Dinner _____/_____

DAY 6

Daily aerobic activity (minutes) _____

Grams of fiber/fat per meal

Breakfast _____/_____   Total grams of fiber eaten _____

Lunch _____/_____   Total grams of fat eaten _____

Snack _____/_____

Dinner _____/_____

DAY 7

Daily aerobic activity (minutes) _____

Grams of fiber/fat per meal

Breakfast _____/_____   Total grams of fiber eaten _____

Lunch _____/_____   Total grams of fat eaten _____

Snack _____/_____

Dinner _____/_____

Week 3: Starting Your Weight-Loss Program

GOALS FOR THE WEEK

- Continue adopting the RAD eating plan, increasing your fiber intake to 30 grams a day.

- If your goals include losing weight, begin your ten-week weight-loss program by limiting the number of calories you take in each day to a target amount.

- Increase your daily amount of intentional walking by another five hundred steps/five minutes, so that you are walking 2,500 steps/ twenty-five minutes per day for six days this week, with one rest day.

Week 3: Overview

NEW: WEIGHT-LOSS TRACK (CALORIE RESTRICTION PHASE)

If you're like many people who weigh more than they'd like to, you've already tried to reduce your weight through one diet approach or another—most likely with mixed success. So let me start by reassuring you of something: Even if you *don't lose a single pound,* you will still be much healthier—and your glucose metabolism will be much improved—by following the strategies outlined in *The Diabetes Reset.* That's because, as I've noted repeatedly, type 2 diabetes has multiple causes, and being overweight is just one of them—albeit a major one. That said, the odds are very good that following these strategies will also result in your weight going down, even if you don't follow the weight-loss strategy outlined here. Our clinical work suggests that you will lose a certain amount of weight simply by eating the foods recommended by the Rural Asian Diet.

At the same time, if you *are* able to lose a modest amount of weight over the next few months, it will represent another significant boost to your glucose metabolism. The benefits of reducing your body weight by 5% to 7% are especially important if you have been diagnosed with elevated fasting blood glucose or have hypertension or a family history of type 2 diabetes and your BMI is over 25 (over 24, if you are of Asian descent). If these factors apply to you, then I strongly urge you to add the Diabetes Reset Weight-Loss Track to your strategy toolbox. It's really two tracks in one—the Healthy Eating Track, which you're already on, combined with a ten-week calorie-restriction regimen, which kicks in now—in Week 3 of the Diabetes Reset Plan.

The goal: Aim for one pound of weight loss per week over the next ten weeks. If this brings you to your overall goal of a 5% to 7% total weight loss, then you can switch to a maintenance program at the end of the ten weeks. If that rate of weight loss isn't enough to reach this overall goal, then continue on after the end of the ten-week Weight-Loss Track until you've lost at least 5% of your starting weight.

To get started: Carefully weigh yourself and note the result on Day 1 of this week's Diabetes Reset calendar. This is your starting weight. Next, select your goal weight. As noted previously, I recommend aiming for a ten-pound weight loss over the next ten weeks and an ultimate goal of a 5% to 7% reduction in body weight, which has been proven to significantly reduce insulin resistance. You can use the At-a-Glance Weight-Loss Chart on page 84 to help figure out how many pounds this would be in your case. Then record your target weight on Day 1 of this week's calendar as well.

SELECT YOUR DAILY GOAL FOR CALORIES CONSUMED. In Strategy Chapter 2, I outlined two alternative calorie goals for losing weight: either a 500-calorie reduction from your normal intake, rounded to the nearest 1,200-, 1,500-, or 1,800-calorie mark—an approach that for men typically means consuming 1,800 calories per day and for women 1,500 calories—or a regimen of 20 to 25 daily calories per kilogram of body weight, as outlined in the sidebar "The Twenty to Twenty-Five Plan: An Alternative Approach to Calorie Restriction," on page 91. Because the RAD eating plan automatically provides a low- to moderate-calorie mix of foods, you'll have a much easier time limiting your calories eating this way than you would otherwise.

BEGIN TRACKING YOUR CALORIES. Because you're already tracking your fat and fiber intake for your RAD eating plan, simply use the RAD food list to note the calorie content of the various foods you consume as well. (You can also download one of the free smartphone calorie-tracking apps listed on page 92.)

WEIGH YOURSELF REGULARLY. Research has shown the more often people on a weight-loss program weigh themselves, the more weight they lose. Aim to weigh yourself daily if possible, recording your weight on your weekly calendar. At week's end, compare your current weight to your starting weight to determine how many pounds you've lost so far.

TIP FOR THE WEEK: *Pay attention to portion size.* If you limit your portion sizes at each meal to slightly less than you're used to eating, while also emphasizing high-fiber, low-fat food choices, your calorie intake will fall into your desired range virtually automatically.

HEALTHY EATING TRACK

Continue to implement the RAD eating plan while tracking your daily fat and fiber intake. As you did last week, keep boosting your daily fiber intake slightly each day until you reach the final RAD target level of 30 grams per day by the end of the week. Make a point of exploring different RAD meal plan options, learning which combinations work best for your palate and your lifestyle.

TIP FOR THE WEEK: *Embrace your power of choice.* As you begin focusing on eating less fat and more fiber, take some time to focus on the wonderful decision-making power that you have now been given. Every decision you make regarding what to eat offers a chance to go for the healthier alternative. As you consider foods you might have eaten without thinking before—a doughnut or potato chips, a fried food, a chicken dish without the skin removed, a soda sweetened with high-fructose corn syrup—realize that this meal or snack offers an opportunity to pick a vegetable, fruit, or whole grain, or a low-fat cheese or meat option, complemented by any number of healthy condiments.

AEROBIC EXERCISE TRACK LEVEL I

The Diabetes Reset Plan calls for a jump of another five hundred steps/five minutes in your daily intentional walking this week, bringing you to 2,500 steps/twenty-five minutes of brisk walking per day for six days this week. This brings you up to Level I in the Diabetes Reset aerobics program: 150 minutes of moderate-intensity aerobic exercise each week, an amount that numerous studies have shown is enough to significantly reduce type 2 diabetes risk and improve glucose control. By this same time, your walking program will already have resulted in a measurable improvement in your insulin resistance as well as your endurance. Continue to look for ways to build walking into your daily routine and monitor your body for any signs of wear and tear.

Note: Next week I'm going to ask you to start your strength training program, so this week is a good time to review the section in Strategy Chapter 3 titled "Resistance Exercise Options: Pros and Cons" on page 124. Consider which strength training approach makes sense for you, and arrange to purchase the needed equipment or gain access to a gym with strength training machines.

TIP FOR THE WEEK: *Having trouble walking?—go recumbent.* If you have pain that makes walking difficult, or if your weight makes exercise difficult, then I strongly advise purchasing a recumbent stationary bike. These bikes, which allow you to recline back in a cushioned seat while using your legs to push on hip-high pedals, are far more comfortable than an upright stationary bike. They also eliminate all stress on your back and don't place pressure on your groin, making it much easier to pedal for an extended period of time. In addition, the armchair-like seat makes it easy to chat with a friend or watch a favorite television show or movie as you work your leg and hip muscles. Healthy exercise doesn't get any more comfortable than this! Many models are available for home use, starting at less than $200. Manufacturers include Nautilus, Marcy, Schwinn, Velocity, Kettler, Sunny Health & Fitness, and FreeMotion.

Diabetes Reset Calendar—Week 3

DAY 1

Daily aerobic activity (minutes) ____

Grams of fiber/fat per meal

Breakfast_____/_____

Lunch_____/_____

Snack _____/_____

Dinner _____/_____

Total grams fiber _____

Total grams fat _____

Total calories _____

Target calories _____

Starting weight _____

Goal weight _____

Current weight _____

DAY 2

Daily aerobic activity (minutes) ____

Grams of fiber/fat per meal

Breakfast_____/_____

Lunch_____/_____

Snack _____/_____

Dinner _____/_____

Total grams fiber _____

Total grams fat _____

Total calories _____

Target calories _____

Current weight _____

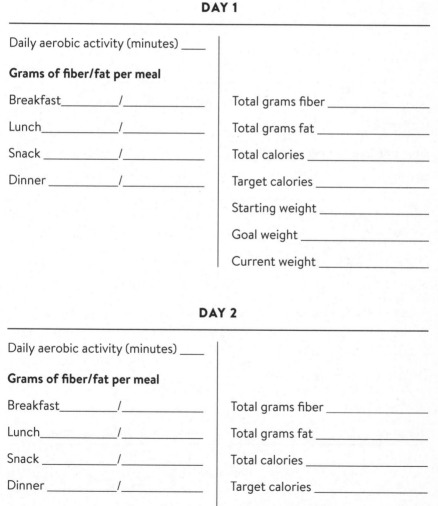

DAY 3

Daily aerobic activity (minutes) _____

Grams of fiber/fat per meal

Breakfast _____/_____   Total grams fiber _____

Lunch _____/_____   Total grams fat _____

Snack _____/_____   Total calories _____

Dinner _____/_____   Target calories _____

                                           Current weight _____

DAY 4

Daily aerobic activity (minutes) _____

Grams of fiber/fat per meal

Breakfast _____/_____   Total grams fiber _____

Lunch _____/_____   Total grams fat _____

Snack _____/_____   Total calories _____

Dinner _____/_____   Target calories _____

                                           Current weight _____

DAY 5

Daily aerobic activity (minutes) _____

Grams of fiber/fat per meal

Breakfast _____/_____   Total grams fiber _____

Lunch _____/_____   Total grams fat _____

Snack _____/_____   Total calories _____

Dinner _____/_____   Target calories _____

                                           Current weight _____

DAY 6

Daily aerobic activity (minutes) _____

Grams of fiber/fat per meal

Breakfast _____/_____   Total grams fiber _____

Lunch _____/_____   Total grams fat _____

Snack _____/_____   Total calories _____

Dinner _____/_____   Target calories _____

                                            Current weight _____

DAY 7

Daily aerobic activity (minutes) _____

Grams of fiber/fat per meal

Breakfast _____/_____   Total grams fiber _____

Lunch _____/_____   Total grams fat _____

Snack _____/_____   Total calories _____

Dinner _____/_____   Target calories _____

                                            Starting weight _____

                                            Goal weight _____

                                            Current weight _____

                                            Pounds lost _____

Week 4: Building Strength

GOALS FOR THE WEEK

- Continue maintaining your RAD eating plan and, if necessary, your ten-week weight-loss plan.

- Continue your walking program of 2,500 steps/twenty-five minutes of brisk walking per day.

- Begin your strength training program by doing one to two resistance workouts this week.

Week 4: Overview

NEW: STRENGTH TRAINING TRACK

The biggest development this week is adding strength training to your exercise routine. Using resistance exercises to increase your strength and muscle mass provides important additional benefits in terms of reducing insulin resistance in your muscles. The section in Strategy Chapter 3 titled "Designing Your Own Strength Training Routine" provides detailed instructions on starting your own strength training program.

For maximum benefits, I recommend doing two strength training sessions each week. If this seems too daunting or time consuming, then begin with just one session—but I strongly urge you to do some resistance training on the major muscle groups of your upper and lower body each week. You'll need to set aside at least a thirty-minute window for each session, which should include eight to ten resistance exercises. (As noted in Week 7, you can also break up your sessions by working some muscle groups one day and the remaining muscle groups on a different day.)

TIP FOR THE WEEK: *Pick your resistance.* Hand weights, resistance tubes or bands, weight machines—they'll all help you build strength and muscle mass, when done properly. You'll need to choose which approach works best for your personality, lifestyle, and environment. If you join a health club or a gym, you'll have weight machines at your disposal, which have easily adjustable weight loads and guide your movements along a preset track. Hand weights (also known as dumbbells) can be bought for use at home, and many gyms have them as well. Resistance tubes or bands can be used virtually anywhere because they fit easily into a briefcase, large handbag, or suitcase.

HEALTHY EATING TRACK

Here in Week 4, a diet focused on high-fiber, low-fat foods should be starting to feel natural (which in fact it is). Continue tracking your daily fiber and fat consumption as you explore which food combinations and meal plans work best for you.

TIP FOR THE WEEK: *Keep the protein, lose the fat.* As you make your protein choices for each meal, emphasize low-fat seafood options, such as broiled fish; and also remove the skin from all poultry; cut away any visible fat from meat; and consume as little processed meat—such as ground beef, hot dogs, bacon, and sausage—as possible. Remember, too, whole grains and legumes eaten in combination make an excellent vegetable-based protein source.

WEIGHT-LOSS TRACK

You're into your second week of weight loss—so far, so good. Continue to track your calorie intake and weigh yourself daily, noting any change from your starting weight at the end of the week. Between your RAD eating plan, your increased physical exercise, and your new calorie-restriction program, you may well find you've already dropped a pound or two from your starting weight. In this second week of your calorie-restriction program, you may also start noticing "trouble spots" where you find yourself chafing at your daily calorie limit. If so, concentrate on finding tasty high-fiber foods that won't add much to your calorie load.

TIP FOR THE WEEK: *Use a calorie-tracking app.* Keeping track of the calories you're consuming with each meal and snack is the only way you can really know if you're properly implementing the Diabetes Reset Weight-Loss Track. Fortunately, tracking calories has never been easier thanks to a number of excellent—and free—smartphone apps. Here are three of the best:

- *Lose it!* (For iPhone and Android) Contains a comprehensive database of foods along with their calories and nutritional content, plus templates that let you calculate calories consumed for each meal as well as calories burned in exercise.

- *MyFitnessPal calorie counter and fitness tracker.* (For iPhone, Android, BlackBerry, and Windows Phone) Includes calorie and nutritional content for more than seven hundred thousand foods, a barcode scanner that analyzes nutritional information of packaged foods, and an exercise calorie calculator.

- *MyNetDiary calorie counter.* (For iPhone and Android phones) Includes calorie and nutrition information for more than four hundred thousand foods, allowing you to log daily meals and workouts.

AEROBIC EXERCISE TRACK LEVEL I

Congratulations on reaching the fourth week of your exercise plan. You're doing a great job ramping up your activity and your fitness level. Continue doing 2,500 steps/twenty-five minutes of brisk walking per day or its equivalent for six days this week. In addition to the short-term boost in insulin sensitivity that exercise provides, the past several weeks of activity have also been improving the function of the mitochondria in the muscles you're using, providing a long-term boost to insulin sensitivity as well.

TIP FOR THE WEEK: *Exercise: The ultimate makeover.* Your muscles never lose their ability to adapt to exercise by increasing their tone and endurance (through aerobic exercise) and their strength (through resistance training). In addition, other parts of your body will adapt along with your muscles—your blood supply, which grows new capillaries to feed your working muscles; your heart, which gradually starts to beat more powerfully; and your muscles' energy system, which becomes better at converting glucose, amino acids, and fatty acids into energy—a key reason why exercise helps prevent and control diabetes. As you exercise each day, take satisfaction in the fact that every minute of activity is changing your body for the better.

Diabetes Reset Calendar—Week 4

DAY 1

Daily aerobic activity (minutes) _____ | Strength workout (yes/no) _____

Grams of fiber/fat per meal

Breakfast _____/_____ | Total grams fiber _____

Lunch _____/_____ | Total grams fat _____

Snack _____/_____ | Total calories _____

Dinner _____/_____ | Target calories _____

| Current weight _____

DAY 2

Daily aerobic activity (minutes) _____ | Strength workout (yes/no) _____

Grams of fiber/fat per meal

Breakfast _____/_____ | Total grams fiber _____

Lunch _____/_____ | Total grams fat _____

Snack _____/_____ | Total calories _____

Dinner _____/_____ | Target calories _____

| Current weight _____

DAY 3

Daily aerobic activity (minutes) _____   Strength workout (yes/no) _____

Grams of fiber/fat per meal

Breakfast _____/_____   Total grams fiber _____

Lunch _____/_____   Total grams fat _____

Snack _____/_____   Total calories _____

Dinner _____/_____   Target calories _____

                                             Current weight _____

DAY 4

Daily aerobic activity (minutes) _____   Strength workout (yes/no) _____

Grams of fiber/fat per meal

Breakfast _____/_____   Total grams fiber _____

Lunch _____/_____   Total grams fat _____

Snack _____/_____   Total calories _____

Dinner _____/_____   Target calories _____

                                             Current weight _____

DAY 5

Daily aerobic activity (minutes) _____   Strength workout (yes/no) _____

Grams of fiber/fat per meal

Breakfast _____/_____   Total grams fiber _____

Lunch _____/_____   Total grams fat _____

Snack _____/_____   Total calories _____

Dinner _____/_____   Target calories _____

                                             Current weight _____

DAY 6

Daily aerobic activity (minutes) ____

Grams of fiber/fat per meal

Breakfast _____ / _____

Lunch _____ / _____

Snack _____ / _____

Dinner _____ / _____

Strength workout (yes/no) _____

Total grams fiber _____

Total grams fat _____

Total calories _____

Target calories _____

Current weight _____

DAY 7

Daily aerobic activity (minutes) ____

Grams of fiber/fat per meal

Breakfast _____ / _____

Lunch _____ / _____

Snack _____ / _____

Dinner _____ / _____

Total grams fiber _____

Strength workout (yes/no) _____

Total grams fat _____

Total calories _____

Target calories _____

Current weight _____

Pounds lost _____

Week 5: Taking Aim at Inflammation

GOALS FOR THE WEEK

- Continue maintaining your RAD eating plan and, if necessary, your ten-week weight-loss plan.

- Continue your walking program of 2,500 steps/twenty-five minutes of brisk walking per day as well as your strength training program of one to two resistance exercise sessions per week.

- Begin taking steps to evaluate and treat any chronic inflammation you might be experiencing.

Week 5: Overview

NEW: INFLAMMATION-FIGHTING TRACK

This week, take an inventory of possible sources of inflammation in your body. If you are losing weight, you're already reducing one important inflammation source. But as Strategy Chapter 5 explains, there are many other potential causes of inflammation as well. If you haven't had your blood levels of C-reactive protein (CRP)—a marker for systemic inflammation—checked recently, I urge you to have this simple and inexpensive blood test done.

TIP FOR THE WEEK: *Take care of your teeth and gums.* Because gum disease is one of the most common types of chronic inflammation—and is also a condition that has been linked to increased diabetes risk—this is an ideal time to review your dental hygiene. You should brush thoroughly twice a day with fluoride toothpaste, being sure to brush along the gum line as well as the surfaces of your teeth, and floss daily. Rinsing with an antibacterial mouthwash after brushing may also help, especially if you have gum disease. In addition, you should see a dentist twice yearly for a cleaning and checkup.

HEALTHY EATING TRACK

In Week 5 of your new eating routine, you should be detecting a noticeable increase in your energy level and feeling of well-being, thanks to the increased nutrients and reduced fats you're consuming. As you implement the RAD eating plan, continue tracking your fiber and fat consumption to make sure you're hitting your daily targets.

TIP FOR THE WEEK: *Branch out on the vegetable front.* This is a perfect time to start exploring different ways to prepare vegetable dishes. Stir-frying in a bit of olive or canola oil; grilling with a low-fat marinade; mixing steamed, stir-fried, or grilled veggies with a cooked whole grain or slow-cooking them with chicken or fish are all great ways to put a flavorful new twist on even the most familiar vegetables.

WEIGHT-LOSS TRACK

Congratulations—you've made it to Week 3 of your calorie-restriction program! If you've been able to stay within your prescribed calorie total each day, give yourself a pat on the back. If your daily calorie totals have been over the limit, continue to track your weight and daily calorie intake while refocusing your efforts.

TIP FOR THE WEEK: *Fight hunger with high-fiber, high-protein snacks.* One of the hardest parts of restricting your calorie intake are those moments when you're hit with a wave of hunger and decide to throw your diet to the winds in favor of a quick fix of high-calorie food. To counter these urges, have some high-fiber, low-fat, low-sugar snacks on hand. The high-fiber content and sheer volume of these foods makes them filling, while their lack of fat and sugar keeps their calorie content low. Try hummus and whole-grain bread, whole-grain cereal with low-fat milk, vegetable soups, steamed green beans or broccoli, raw carrots or celery, a baked sweet potato, a banana, or an apple. To further quench your hunger pangs, add some lean protein such as skinless chicken, hardboiled egg whites, or low-fat yogurt (for additional fiber, add blueberries, strawberries, or banana).

AEROBIC EXERCISE TRACK LEVEL I

You should be feeling stronger than ever during your aerobic sessions now, as you get over any initial feelings of fatigue from your new level of daily physical activity. This week, concentrate on managing your schedule to fit in your daily walking total of 2,500 steps/twenty-five minutes per day over six days. If time pressures are causing you to skip a session here or there, work on finding alternative time slots during the day.

TIP FOR THE WEEK: *Partner power.* Research has shown that social support is an important factor in maintaining a program of regular exercise: As you settle into your more active lifestyle, seek out some walking partners to join you for sessions of brisk walking in the morning, over the lunch hour, or at the workday's end. This is also a good time to think about joining a walking club or some other group that meets regularly for aerobic exercise sessions.

STRENGTH TRAINING TRACK

Continue to do a full group of strength training exercises one to two days this week. You may experience some muscle soreness in the second week of your resistance exercise program. If so, then switch to a lighter resistance level and do very easy repetitions of each exercise until the soreness subsides.

TIP FOR THE WEEK: *Succeeding by failing.* The key to building strength is to exhaust your muscles' short-term energy supply, which means working them to their limit within the space of a minute or two. In practice, that requires doing each resistance exercise ten to fifteen times with a heavy enough resistance that your muscles are starting to fail (tire to the point where they can no longer lift the weight) by the time you reach the final "lift" or movement—meaning that this last repetition should be fairly difficult to complete. If you feel as if you could easily do several more repetitions following repetition number fifteen, then the resistance you're using is not heavy enough.

Diabetes Reset Calendar—Week 5

DAY 1

Daily aerobic activity (minutes) _____	Strength workout (yes/no) _____
Grams of fiber/fat per meal	
Breakfast _____/_____	Total grams fiber _____
Lunch _____/_____	Total grams fat _____
Snack _____/_____	Total calories _____
Dinner _____/_____	Target calories _____
	Current weight _____

DAY 2

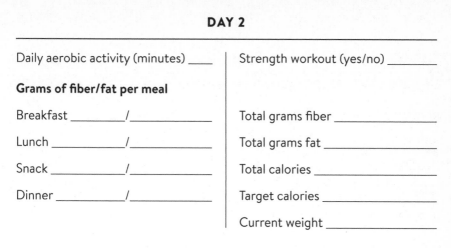

Daily aerobic activity (minutes) _____ | Strength workout (yes/no) _____

Grams of fiber/fat per meal

Breakfast _____/_____ | Total grams fiber _____

Lunch _____/_____ | Total grams fat _____

Snack _____/_____ | Total calories _____

Dinner _____/_____ | Target calories _____

     | Current weight _____

DAY 3

Daily aerobic activity (minutes) _____ | Strength workout (yes/no) _____

Grams of fiber/fat per meal

Breakfast _____/_____ | Total grams fiber _____

Lunch _____/_____ | Total grams fat _____

Snack _____/_____ | Total calories _____

Dinner _____/_____ | Target calories _____

     | Current weight _____

DAY 4

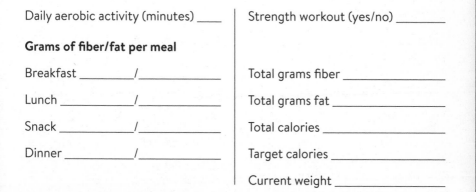

Daily aerobic activity (minutes) _____ | Strength workout (yes/no) _____

Grams of fiber/fat per meal

Breakfast _____/_____ | Total grams fiber _____

Lunch _____/_____ | Total grams fat _____

Snack _____/_____ | Total calories _____

Dinner _____/_____ | Target calories _____

     | Current weight _____

DAY 5

Daily aerobic activity (minutes) _____   Strength workout (yes/no) _____

Grams of fiber/fat per meal

Breakfast _____/_____   Total grams fiber _____

Lunch _____/_____   Total grams fat _____

Snack _____/_____   Total calories _____

Dinner _____/_____   Target calories _____

                                           Current weight _____

DAY 6

Daily aerobic activity (minutes) _____   Strength workout (yes/no) _____

Grams of fiber/fat per meal

Breakfast _____/_____   Total grams fiber _____

Lunch _____/_____   Total grams fat _____

Snack _____/_____   Total calories _____

Dinner _____/_____   Target calories _____

                                           Current weight _____

DAY 7

Daily aerobic activity (minutes) _____   Strength workout (yes/no) _____

Grams of fiber/fat per meal

Breakfast _____/_____   Total grams fiber _____

Lunch _____/_____   Total grams fat _____

Snack _____/_____   Total calories _____

Dinner _____/_____   Target calories _____

                                           Starting weight _____

                                           Goal weight _____

                                           Current weight _____

                                           Pounds lost _____

Week 6: Improving Your Sleep

GOALS FOR THE WEEK

- Continue maintaining your RAD eating plan and, if necessary, your ten-week weight-loss plan.

- Continue your walking program of 2,500 steps/twenty-five minutes of brisk walking per day as well as your strength training program of one to two resistance exercise sessions per week.

- Begin taking steps to evaluate and treat any sleep problems that may be interfering with your ability to get a full, restful night's sleep on a regular basis.

Week 6: Overview

NEW: HEALTHY SLEEP TRACK

Begin this week by addressing any sleep issues you are having. Your diet and exercise program may already be helping you to get more restful sleep at night, but if you are continuing to have trouble falling or staying asleep, or if you wake up feeling tired, then I urge you to carefully reread Strategy Chapter 6 and try the techniques described there. As part of this strategy, you can start tracking your nightly sleep on your weekly calendar.

TIP FOR THE WEEK: *Let darkness reign.* Melatonin is a hormone produced by your body that plays a key role in regulating your sleep cycle. Because your body's pineal gland produces this chemical only in the absence of light, maintaining a dark sleeping environment is critical, especially if you tend to have difficulty falling asleep or often wake up in the night and can't back to sleep. Make sure you have light-blocking shades or curtains over your windows, and cover up any glowing electrical devices such as clocks or cable TV boxes. In addition, for an hour or so before going to bed, dim your lights and avoid watching television or looking at your computer screen.

HEALTHY EATING TRACK

As you approach the halfway point of the Diabetes Reset Healthy Eating Track, you should be feeling a new sense of energy and well-being from your new eating pattern. Continue to implement the RAD eating plan while tracking your daily fiber and fat consumption. Make special note of the meal plans that seem to be working well for you in terms of preparation, enjoyment, and satiety.

TIP FOR THE WEEK: *For healthy fats, make them mono.* Where a healthy diet is concerned, you should not only watch how much fat you eat, but what kind. Chemically altered trans-fats are the unhealthiest fat type of all and are in the process of being phased out in the U.S. Saturated fats (so-called because their chemical structure contains the maximum possible number of hydrogen atoms, meaning they are "saturated" with hydrogen) are also clearly damaging to your cardiovascular system and your glucose metabolism. Saturated fat is found mainly in milk products, red meat, and poultry. On the other hand, there's evidence that unsaturated fat, which is found in plants and contains fewer hydrogen atoms, can actually improve cholesterol levels, insulin response, and glucose control. The healthiest type of unsaturated fat appears to be monounsaturated fat, which increases satiety compared to saturated fat and may also help reduce dangerous abdominal fat—in part by boosting your metabolic rate. Some of the best sources of monounsaturated fat are olive oil, canola oil, peanut oil, and safflower oil. Use moderate amounts of these oils whenever you use oil to cook or make a salad dressing. Other sources include fish, avocados, nuts, and seeds.

WEIGHT-LOSS TRACK

Here in Week 4 of your weight-loss program, you should be seeing at least a slight drop in your weight. If so, congratulations! If not, then this is a time to reevaluate your daily eating and exercise patterns. If you are having difficulty sticking to your daily calorie count, look for areas where you can substitute more high-fiber, low-calorie foods for what you're currently eating. Meanwhile, continue to track your daily calorie intake and your weight.

TIP FOR THE WEEK: *Start the day with a high-fiber breakfast.* Data show that eating a breakfast that includes a high-fiber cereal is extremely common among people who are successful at losing weight. Look for whole-grain cereals, particularly those that contain 100% bran or close to it. Add fat-free milk and top it with bananas, blueberries, strawberries, or raspberries or eat some fruit on the side, and you have a perfect high-fiber, low-fat breakfast that will leave you feeling full and energized for hours afterward. If you're still hungry, add a slice of whole-grain toast with a fat-free butter substitute or some scrambled or hard-boiled egg whites.

AEROBIC EXERCISE TRACK LEVEL I

By now your body will have largely adapted to your new program of 2,500 steps/twenty-five minutes of brisk walking per day (or its equivalent). If you can maintain this level of exercise into the future, you'll be doing one of the most important things possible to improve your glucose control and keep type 2 diabetes from occurring or progressing.

Next week, for those who want to lower the risk even further, I'll address the option of taking your aerobic exercise program to the next level.

TIP FOR THE WEEK: *Pamper yourself.* If you're not used to daily exercise, you may feel a little fatigued or sore as your body adjusts to the new demands you're placing on it. Repay your body by pampering it this week. Take a relaxing hot bath or treat yourself to a massage. And be sure to get plenty of restful sleep, which is especially important right now as your body ramps up its aerobic capabilities.

STRENGTH TRAINING TRACK

Here in Week 3 of your strength training program, your muscles should be starting to adapt to the new challenges you've been giving them—in fact, you may even be noticing some increased tone in your arms and legs. Continue to do a full group of strength training exercises one to two days a week. If the weight you're lifting is starting to feel easy by the last repetition of each set, then it's time to increase the resistance slightly.

TIP FOR THE WEEK: *A different "forty-eight-hour rule."* In Strategy Chapter 3, I explained how the insulin-sensitizing effect of aerobic exercise lasts forty-eight hours, which is why you should try not to allow more than forty-eight hours to elapse between aerobic sessions. Although weight training has a similar insulin-sensitizing effect, it carries a different rule, which says you should always wait at least forty-eight hours between workouts for a given muscle group. The reason: Because you are working your muscle fibers intensively with strength training, they require that much time to fully recover before your next weight-lifting session.

INFLAMMATION-FIGHTING TRACK

Continue to develop your inflammation-fighting strategy by seeking treatment for any inflammatory conditions and adding anti-inflammatory foods and herbs to your daily menu.

TIP FOR THE WEEK: *Know your CRP level.* If you haven't had your blood levels of C-reactive protein (CRP) checked recently, ask your doctor about getting tested for this marker of general inflammation levels in the body. A CRP reading under 1 milligram per liter (mg/L) is considered normal, indicating a low risk for insulin resistance and heart attack, whereas 1 mg/L to 3 mg/L has been associated with an elevated risk of insulin resistance, and a level above 3 mg/L is associated with high risk of insulin resistance.

Diabetes Reset Calendar—Week 6

DAY 1

Daily aerobic activity (minutes) ____

Strength workout (yes/no) _____

Hours slept _____

Daily food totals

Total grams fiber _____

Total grams fat _____

Total calories _____

Target calories _____

Current weight _____

DAY 2

Daily aerobic activity (minutes) ____

Strength workout (yes/no) _____

Hours slept _____

Daily food totals

Total grams fiber _____

Total grams fat _____

Total calories _____

Target calories _____

Current weight _____

DAY 3

Daily aerobic activity (minutes) ____

Strength workout (yes/no) _____

Hours slept _____

Daily food totals

Total grams fiber _____

Total grams fat _____

Total calories _____

Target calories _____

Current weight _____

DAY 4

Daily aerobic activity (minutes) _____

Strength workout (yes/no) _____

Hours slept _____

Daily food totals

Total grams fiber _____

Total grams fat _____

Total calories _____

Target calories _____

Current weight _____

DAY 5

Daily aerobic activity (minutes) _____

Strength workout (yes/no) _____

Hours slept _____

Daily food totals

Total grams fiber _____

Total grams fat _____

Total calories _____

Target calories _____

Current weight _____

DAY 6

Daily aerobic activity (minutes) _____

Strength workout (yes/no) _____

Hours slept _____

Daily food totals

Total grams fiber _____

Total grams fat _____

Total calories _____

Target calories _____

Current weight _____

DAY 7

Daily aerobic activity (minutes) ____	**Daily food totals**
Strength workout (yes/no) _____	Total grams fiber _____
Hours slept _____	Total grams fat _____
	Total calories _____
	Target calories _____
	Starting weight _____
	Goal weight _____
	Current weight _____
	Pounds lost _____

Week 7: Upping Your Aerobic Program to the Next Level (Optional)

GOALS FOR THE WEEK

- Continue maintaining your RAD eating plan and, if necessary, your ten-week weight-loss plan.

- Aerobic Exercise Track Level I: Continue your walking program of 2,500 steps/twenty-five minutes of brisk walking per day.

- Aerobic Exercise Track Level II (optional): Increase your aerobic activity level by adding five additional minutes per day for a daily total of thirty minutes of brisk walking or other moderate-intensity aerobic exercise.

- Continue your strength training program of one to two resistance exercise sessions per week.

- Continue your anti-inflammatory and healthy sleeping strategies.

Week 7: Overview

GLUCOSE CHECK 2

During this week, pick two days and use a blood glucose home test kit to check your blood glucose levels four times on each of those days—when you first wake up, and then again one hour after each meal. Compare these sets of readings and their average to your first set of glucose readings. Ideally, you'll see a noticeable improvement over the past six weeks.

NEW: AEROBIC EXERCISE TRACK LEVELS I AND II

Now that you've reached Level I in the Diabetes Reset Aerobic Exercise Track of 2,500 steps/twenty-five minutes brisk walking per day plus 5,000 steps per day of incidental walking, you're at a level of activity that equates to a significantly reduced risk for prediabetes and diabetes, as well as heart attack, stroke, and other cardiovascular conditions.

If you simply stay at this level, you will continue to see steady improvements in your fitness and your glucose metabolism. If, however, you can double your amount of moderate-intensity aerobic exercise to Level II—fifty minutes per day, six days a week, for a total of three hundred minutes per week—you will lower your diabetes risk and improve your glucose metabolism even further. This halfway point in your Diabetes Reset Plan is an opportune time to begin increasing your daily aerobic activity by adding additional brisk walking or by branching out into a different aerobic sport such as cycling, jogging, swimming, riding a stationary bike, or an equivalent activity. Simply follow the scheduled weekly increases of five minutes total aerobic activity per day until you reach a level you're comfortable with.

If you decide you're ready to increase your daily activity level, then your goal this week is to do thirty minutes of moderate-intensity aerobic exercise—either brisk walking or its equivalent—for six days this week, with one rest day.

TIP FOR THE WEEK: *Consider cross-training.* Dividing your exercise session among two or more types of physical activity is beneficial—it's more interesting, and it works different muscles while still providing all the cardio you need. Combining different aerobic activities, an approach known as cross-training, has other benefits as well: By building endurance in different muscle groups, cross-training stimulates the diabetes-fighting effects of exercise in more of your skeletal muscles. It also lessens the risk of an overuse injury by spreading wear and tear among a wider range of bones, joints, and connective tissue. Plus, it's enjoyable to have options: Switching between a brisk walk one day and an invigorating bicycle ride the next, or even combining each activity in a single day's exercise, provides varied challenges and experiences and keeps boredom at bay. If you do decide to cross-train, try to do each activity at least every forty-eight hours to gain the full insulin-enhancing benefits of that activity and to maintain your endurance in that set of muscles.

HEALTHY EATING TRACK

Continue to implement the RAD eating plan while tracking your daily fiber and fat consumption. While noting which menu items are working well, don't stop exploring the different alternatives described in the RAD meal plan options—both to keep your eating plan interesting and to see which meal plans fit your lifestyle best.

TIP FOR THE WEEK: *The colors of health.* The different shades found in various vegetables, fruits, grains, and legumes are the result of the many different bioflavonoids (health-promoting micronutrients) that each plant type contains. The more varied the colors of the plant foods you eat, the greater the range of bioflavonoids—and health benefits—you'll get.

WEIGHT-LOSS TRACK

If you are continuing to see a small but steady weight loss, keep up the good work! If not, there's no need to despair. You are already improving your health significantly through eating a healthier diet, increasing your physical activity, and following the other Diabetes Reset strategies. Rather than trying to cut your daily calories further, continue to look for ways to increase the amount of fiber and complex carbs you're eating while decreasing fat and added sugar. By making you feel satiated after eating, this approach will naturally make it easier to stick to your daily calorie goal.

TIP FOR THE WEEK: *Cultivate your assertive side.* When pursuing a weight-loss program, sticking to your guns is essential. If your family or friends aren't being as supportive as they could be, practice the basics of assertive behavior by politely but firmly indicating what your needs are and asking for help in getting those needs met. For example, you might say, "Let's try a place with a salad bar rather than the usual burger joint tonight, because it has food choices that fit better with my diet."

STRENGTH TRAINING TRACK

Continue to do a full group of strength training exercises one to two days this week. Consider adding a second weekly session at this point to increase the benefits to your glucose metabolism.

TIP FOR THE WEEK: *Divide and conquer.* If you're finding it hard to set aside the half hour needed to do eight or ten strength training exercises for various muscle groups, try doing different parts of your strength training on different days. For example, you could do all of your upper-body strength exercises one day and all of your lower-body exercises the following day. Just be sure to wait at least forty-eight hours between resistance exercises for any specific muscle group to give it time to recover.

INFLAMMATION-FIGHTING TRACK

Continue to develop your inflammation-fighting strategy by seeking treatment for any inflammatory conditions and adding anti-inflammatory foods and herbs to your daily menu.

TIP FOR THE WEEK: *Foods that fight inflammation.* If inflammation is an issue for you, make a point of including the following inflammation-fighting foods in your RAD eating plan: fish high in healthful omega-3 fats (salmon, tuna, sardines, mackerel, herring), colorful fruits (raspberries, blueberries), cruciferous vegetables (broccoli, Brussels sprouts, cauliflower), mushrooms, nuts, legumes, soy and soy products, garlic, onions, and green or black tea.

HEALTHY SLEEP TRACK

Continue taking steps to address any issues that are preventing you from getting seven to eight hours of restful sleep each night. If that goal is still elusive, review your daily schedule to see if you're leaving enough time for sleeping. Not only will better sleep help your glucose metabolism, but it will improve your general health and stress levels as well.

TIP FOR THE WEEK: *Take a hot bath two hours before bedtime.* If you raise your body temperature by soaking in a hot bath a couple of hours before retiring, you'll trigger a "rebound" drop in body temperature one to two hours later. Because sleep is associated with a slightly lower body temperature, this will make it easier to fall asleep.

Diabetes Reset Calendar—Week 7

DAY 1

Daily aerobic activity (minutes) ____	**Daily food totals**
Strength workout (yes/no) _____	Total grams fiber _____
Hours slept _____	Total grams fat _____
	Total calories _____
	Target calories _____
	Current weight _____

DAY 2

Daily aerobic activity (minutes) _____

Strength workout (yes/no) _____

Hours slept _____

Daily food totals

Total grams fiber _____

Total grams fat _____

Total calories _____

Target calories _____

Current weight _____

DAY 3

Daily aerobic activity (minutes) _____

Strength workout (yes/no) _____

Hours slept _____

Daily food totals

Total grams fiber _____

Total grams fat _____

Total calories _____

Target calories _____

Current weight _____

DAY 4

Daily aerobic activity (minutes) _____

Strength workout (yes/no) _____

Hours slept _____

Daily food totals

Total grams fiber _____

Total grams fat _____

Total calories _____

Target calories _____

Current weight _____

DAY 5

Daily aerobic activity (minutes) _____

Strength workout (yes/no) _____

Hours slept _____

Daily food totals

Total grams fiber _____

Total grams fat _____

Total calories _____

Target calories _____

Current weight _____

DAY 6

Daily aerobic activity (minutes) _____

Strength workout (yes/no) _____

Hours slept _____

Daily food totals

Total grams fiber _____

Total grams fat _____

Total calories _____

Target calories _____

Current weight _____

DAY 7

Daily aerobic activity (minutes) _____

Strength workout (yes/no) _____

Hours slept _____

Daily food totals

Total grams fiber _____

Total grams fat _____

Total calories _____

Target calories _____

Starting weight _____

Goal weight _____

Current weight _____

Pounds lost _____

Week 8: Addressing Your Stress

GOALS FOR THE WEEK

- Continue maintaining your RAD eating plan and, if necessary, your ten-week weight-loss plan.

- Aerobic Exercise Track Level I: Continue your walking program of 2,500 steps/twenty-five minutes of brisk walking per day, with one rest day per week.

- Aerobic Exercise Track Level II: Either maintain your current activity level or add five additional minutes per day for a daily total of thirty-five minutes of brisk walking or other moderate-intensity aerobic exercise, with one rest day per week.

- Continue your strength training program of one to two resistance exercise sessions per week.

- Continue your anti-inflammatory and healthy sleeping strategies.

- Assess your stress level and potential sources of stress in your life, and then start developing a strategy to manage chronic stressors.

Week 8: Overview

NEW: ANTI-STRESS TRACK

This week, I want you to turn your focus to Strategy Chapter 7 of *The Diabetes Reset,* which discusses how chronic stress can affect your glucose metabolism and describes various approaches to stress reduction. Take a few minutes to review the list of chronic stress symptoms in the tip that follows. If you think these may apply to you, then consider trying the stress-reduction techniques in Chapter 7. Give each approach at least a few days to work. If it doesn't seem to have a calming effect, then drop it and try another. As you try different stress-reduction strategies, carefully note which ones appear to work best for you.

TIP FOR THE WEEK: *Know the signs of chronic stress.* Signs of stress may include: feeling tired or fatigued for no clear reason; problems falling or staying asleep; difficulty concentrating; memory lapses; unexplained irritability; feelings of nervousness, anxiety or sadness; being consistently angry for no clear reason; recurring chest pain, headaches, backaches or muscle pain; gastrointestinal upset; lack of interest in activities you usually enjoy; restlessness; inability to relax; compulsive eating; and excessive consumption of alcohol.

HEALTHY EATING TRACK

Continue to implement the RAD eating plan while tracking your daily fiber and fat consumption. This is a good time to check in with family and friends to ask for some suggestions on meal plans and preparation ideas.

TIP FOR THE WEEK: *Eat smaller meals, more often.* If you have been diagnosed with prediabetes or type 2 diabetes, it's important not to eat too much at a time or eat too quickly. Reason: This will cause your blood glucose levels to rise more sharply, putting additional strain on an already impaired glucose metabolism. Whether or not you're on the Diabetes Reset Weight-Loss Track right now, I recommend eating normal portion sizes of all servings at every meal—3.5 ounces of animal protein, as well as a half cup each of vegetables, legumes, grains, and fruits—and chewing each mouthful of food at least ten times before swallowing.

If you find you're still hungry after eating a reasonably sized meal, simply have another small meal a couple of hours later. Although this may seem inconvenient, you'll be protecting your pancreas from a glucose overload—a trade-off that's well worth it.

WEIGHT-LOSS TRACK

At six weeks into your weight-loss program, you should have a good sense of how it's progressing. If you haven't lost weight or have plateaued in your weight loss, don't be discouraged. Your new eating patterns and increased physical activity have set the stage for healthy weight loss. Instead, look hard at your daily eating patterns to identify sources of excess calories and work on eliminating these sources over the next several weeks.

TIP FOR THE WEEK: *Keep your eyes on the prize.* Losing weight is never easy—but any amount of weight loss, even a few pounds, will help improve your glucose control. Remember that you will be reaching your weight-loss goal as long as you're able to lose at least 5% of your weight by the end of your weight-loss program. That's just 12.5 pounds, if you currently weigh 250. And of course, you're improving your health and glucose metabolism by following your Diabetes Reset strategies, *whether or not* you reach your weight-loss goal.

AEROBIC EXERCISE TRACK LEVELS I AND II

Level I exercisers, stay on course: At this point, your routine is hopefully becoming second nature—a good sign!

Level II exercisers, you have the option this week of staying at thirty minutes per week or increasing your daily aerobic activity by another five minutes, to thirty-five minutes per day, six days a week, with one rest day. If you feel any soreness or excessive fatigue, cut back on your activity level until you feel fresh and pain-free.

TIP FOR THE WEEK: *Stretch it out.* If you haven't begun stretching already, this is a good time to begin doing a few minutes of gentle stretching at the end of each aerobic session to keep your muscles at an optimal length and ensure a fluid range of motion as you move. Start with the five stretches described on page 135.

STRENGTH TRAINING TRACK

Continue to do a full group of strength training exercises for one to two days this week. Review the amount of weight you're using—increasing it slightly if your last repetitions are feeling too easy for a given exercise.

TIP FOR THE WEEK: *Slower lifting builds stronger muscles.* Although it may be tempting to do resistance exercises as quickly as possible in order to finish each set of repetitions sooner, you'll get better results by lifting at a fairly slow tempo—thereby putting the muscle fibers under tension for a longer period of time. Concentrate on taking several seconds to complete the "lifting" part of each repetition (in which you're pushing or pulling against the weight) in a smooth, controlled fashion, then return to your starting position in the same slow, controlled manner.

INFLAMMATION-FIGHTING TRACK

Continue to develop your inflammation-fighting strategy by seeking treatment for any inflammatory conditions and adding anti-inflammatory foods and herbs to your daily menu.

TIP FOR THE WEEK: *Inflammation check.* If you suffer from recurring ear or sinus infections or asthma, or have an inflammatory autoimmune condition such as psoriasis, celiac or Crohn's disease, or colitis, now is a good time to discuss a serious treatment plan with your doctor. These conditions can affect your body's ability to respond to insulin and may also be damaging your pancreas.

HEALTHY SLEEP TRACK

Continue taking steps to address any issues that are preventing you from getting seven to eight hours of restful sleep each night.

TIP FOR THE WEEK: *Try to wake at the same time each morning, including weekends.* Doing this will help train your body's daily rhythm, enabling you to fall asleep more easily and sleep more soundly throughout the night.

Diabetes Reset Calendar—Week 8

DAY 1

Daily aerobic activity (minutes) ____

Strength workout (yes/no) _____

Hours slept _____

Daily food totals

Total grams fiber _____

Total grams fat _____

Total calories _____

Target calories _____

Current weight _____

DAY 2

Daily aerobic activity (minutes) ____

Strength workout (yes/no) _____

Hours slept _____

Daily food totals

Total grams fiber _____

Total grams fat _____

Total calories _____

Target calories _____

Current weight _____

DAY 3

Daily aerobic activity (minutes) ____

Strength workout (yes/no) _____

Hours slept _____

Daily food totals

Total grams fiber _____

Total grams fat _____

Total calories _____

Target calories _____

Current weight _____

DAY 4

Daily aerobic activity (minutes) _____

Strength workout (yes/no) _____

Hours slept _____

Daily food totals

Total grams fiber _____

Total grams fat _____

Total calories _____

Target calories _____

Current weight _____

DAY 5

Daily aerobic activity (minutes) _____

Strength workout (yes/no) _____

Hours slept _____

Daily food totals

Total grams fiber _____

Total grams fat _____

Total calories _____

Target calories _____

Current weight _____

DAY 6

Daily aerobic activity (minutes) _____

Strength workout (yes/no) _____

Hours slept _____

Daily food totals

Total grams fiber _____

Total grams fat _____

Total calories _____

Target calories _____

Current weight _____

DAY 7

Daily aerobic activity (minutes) ____	**Daily food totals**
Strength workout (yes/no) _____	Total grams fiber _____
Hours slept _____	Total grams fat _____
	Total calories _____
	Target calories _____
	Starting weight _____
	Goal weight _____
	Current weight _____
	Pounds lost _____

Week 9: Activating Your Body's Antioxidants

GOALS FOR THE WEEK

- Continue maintaining your RAD eating plan and, if necessary, your ten-week weight-loss plan.

- Aerobic Exercise Track Level I: Continue your walking program of 2,500 steps/twenty-five minutes of brisk walking per day, with one rest day per week.

- Aerobic Exercise Track Level II: Either maintain your current activity level or add five additional minutes per day for a daily total of forty minutes of brisk walking or other moderate-intensity aerobic exercise, with one rest day per week.

- Continue your strength training program of two resistance exercise sessions per week.

- Continue your anti-inflammatory, healthy sleeping, and stress management strategies.

- Start reducing oxidative stress by adding Phase 2 antioxidant sources to your daily menu.

Week 9: Overview

NEW: NATURAL ANTIOXIDANTS TRACK

This week, the Diabetes Reset Plan sets another important strategy in motion—boosting your body's production of natural antioxidants in order to minimize the negative impact of oxidative stress on your glucose metabolism. As described in Strategy Chapter 8, research suggests this oxidative stress can be combated most effectively by using activating substances called Phase 2 antioxidants to boost production of your body's many different natural antioxidants on the cellular level.

TIP FOR THE WEEK: *Beef up your diet with natural antioxidant-boosting foods.* Begin adding plant foods that are rich in Phase 2 antioxidants to your RAD eating plan. These include cruciferous vegetables (broccoli, broccoli sprouts, Brussels sprouts, cauliflower, and cabbage), salmon, tuna, sardines, mackerel, herring, green tea, coffee, and strawberries.

HEALTHY EATING TRACK

Continue to implement the RAD eating plan while tracking your daily fiber and fat consumption.

TIP FOR THE WEEK: *Skip the sugar and forego the fructose.* As noted in Strategy Chapter 1, I don't agree that all of our nation's diet-related health problems can be traced to the consumption of sugar (actually sucrose, which is half glucose and half fructose) and high-fructose corn sweetener (similar to sucrose, but with slightly more fructose than glucose). That said, however, there's no question that these two food additives are certainly not good for you. They are essentially empty calories, with no nutritional value beyond their ability to provide energy; they promote weight gain by making it easy to overconsume calories because their satiety effect is low (especially when added to sweetened beverages, which the brain registers as much less filling than solid food), and the fructose in them is converted by the liver into fatty acids, contributing to insulin resistance in much the same way that dietary fat does. For these reasons, I strongly recommend being a careful label reader and consuming as little sucrose or high-fructose corn syrup as possible. Eating a diet high in complex carbohydrates will help in this endeavor.

WEIGHT-LOSS TRACK

This is Week 7 of your weight-loss program—a time to stay centered and focused on your goals. If your second blood glucose check was an improvement over the first reading, then any weight you've lost to date has undoubtedly contributed to this.

TIP FOR THE WEEK: *Make peace with your inner child—and parent.* Watch for your own instinctive childlike responses to calorie restriction—rebelling by sneaking extra calories, giving up in anger, or going along with the program while harboring a simmering resentment—and also for your "inner parent" reactions, such as expecting perfection, berating yourself for going over your daily calorie limit, and comparing yourself with others. If you do fall off your diet, instead of getting upset, analyze what caused you to backslide and then address this cause as you calmly resume your program.

AEROBIC EXERCISE TRACK LEVELS I AND II

Level I exercisers, continue your current program. Level II exercisers, you have the option this week of staying at your current activity level or increasing your daily aerobic activity by another five minutes, to forty minutes per day, six days a week, with one rest day.

TIP FOR THE WEEK: *The telltale heartbeat.* One effect of regular aerobic exercise is that your heart gradually adapts by pumping more blood each time it contracts. The result is that your resting heartbeat will start to slow down as you become more fit. If you take a moment before getting out of bed each morning to count your heart beats in one minute, you'll start to see your resting pulse rate get lower—a sign that your exercise routine is paying off.

STRENGTH TRAINING TRACK

Continue to do a full group of strength training exercises one or, if possible, two days a week. If the level of resistance you are using is starting to feel too easy by the last repetition of each set, then it's time to increase the resistance slightly.

TIP FOR THE WEEK: *Are three weekly strength workouts better than two?* Research suggests that doing resistance exercises one day per week is enough to produce significant gains in strength and mass over time. There is also good evidence that doing strength training twice a week builds strength and mass more quickly. Is it worth taking the next step and moving to three strength workouts per week? For the average time-pressed person, the answer is—probably not. Three resistance sessions will produce even faster results, but the difference isn't that dramatic: Some studies have found it yields strength gains of only an additional 15% compared to twice-weekly training.

INFLAMMATION-FIGHTING TRACK

Continue to develop your inflammation-fighting strategy by seeking medical treatment for any chronic inflammatory conditions and adding anti-inflammatory foods and herbs to your daily menu.

HEALTHY SLEEP TRACK

Continue taking steps to address any issues that are preventing you from getting seven to eight hours of restful sleep each night.

ANTI-STRESS TRACK

As you continue to focus on potential stress management strategies, keep in mind that you are already engaging in one of the most effective stress-reduction techniques: regular physical exercise. If you are having success with your sleep-enhancing strategies, that should also help reduce your stress levels. At week's end, write down which strategies you've been trying—and the results—in a notebook or journal, so you can track your progress.

TIP FOR THE WEEK: *Identifying your stressors.* There are some causes of stress that you may be able to address—such as a peripheral relationship that is problematic or time management skills that need improving. Other sources of stress may be less easily changed, such as a job you dislike or conflict with your spouse—but by recognizing the situation as stressful, you can begin strategizing about how to improve it and can also be on guard to the effect it's having on you. With stressful situations that can't be changed, such as dealing with the loss of a loved one, recognizing the stress you are under can help spur you to seek counseling or other forms of support.

Diabetes Reset Calendar—Week 9

DAY 1

Daily aerobic activity (minutes) _____

Strength workout (yes/no) _____

Hours slept _____

Daily food totals

Total grams fiber _____

Total grams fat _____

Total calories _____

Target calories _____

Current weight _____

DAY 2

Daily aerobic activity (minutes) _____

Strength workout (yes/no) _____

Hours slept _____

Daily food totals

Total grams fiber _____

Total grams fat _____

Total calories _____

Target calories _____

Current weight _____

DAY 3

Daily aerobic activity (minutes) _____

Strength workout (yes/no) _____

Hours slept _____

Daily food totals

Total grams fiber _____

Total grams fat _____

Total calories _____

Target calories _____

Current weight _____

DAY 4

Daily aerobic activity (minutes) _____

Strength workout (yes/no) _____

Hours slept _____

Daily food totals

Total grams fiber _____

Total grams fat _____

Total calories _____

Target calories _____

Current weight _____

DAY 5

Daily aerobic activity (minutes) _____

Strength workout (yes/no) _____

Hours slept _____

Daily food totals

Total grams fiber _____

Total grams fat _____

Total calories _____

Target calories _____

Current weight _____

DAY 6

Daily aerobic activity (minutes) ____

Strength workout (yes/no) _____

Hours slept _____

Daily food totals

Total grams fiber _____

Total grams fat _____

Total calories _____

Target calories _____

Current weight _____

DAY 7

Daily aerobic activity (minutes) ____

Strength workout (yes/no) _____

Hours slept _____

Daily food totals

Total grams fiber _____

Total grams fat _____

Total calories _____

Target calories _____

Starting weight _____

Goal weight _____

Current weight _____

Pounds lost _____

Week 10: Bringing Your Brown Fat into Play

GOALS FOR THE WEEK

- Continue maintaining your RAD eating plan and, if necessary, your ten-week weight-loss plan.

- Aerobic Exercise Track Level I: Continue your walking program of 2,500 steps/twenty-five minutes of brisk walking per day, with one rest day per week.

- Aerobic Exercise Track Level II: Either maintain your current activity level or add five additional minutes per day for a daily total of forty-five minutes of brisk walking or other moderate-intensity aerobic exercise, with one rest day per week.

- Continue your strength training program of two resistance exercise sessions per week.

- Continue your anti-inflammatory, healthy sleeping, stress management, and natural antioxidant strategies.

- Begin looking for opportunities to activate your brown fat stores on a daily basis.

Week 10: Overview

NEW: BROWN FAT ACTIVATION TRACK

This week, I'm going to recommend that you explore ways to activate your brown fat stores. The key, as discussed in Strategy Chapter 4, is to keep your environment at a temperature slightly under 70°F for an extended time each day, particularly your neck area, and especially while exercising.

TIP FOR THE WEEK: *Maintaining your cool.* To activate your brown fat on an ongoing basis, search out a sub-70°F environment that you can spend time in each day. If you live in a place that experiences cold winter weather, then spending an hour or more outdoors each day during the winter months—and keeping your neck and collarbone area exposed as you do—will do the trick. Lowering your home thermostat into the mid-60s range will help as well.

HEALTHY EATING TRACK

Continue to implement the RAD eating plan while tracking your daily fiber and fat consumption, using the RAD meal plan options and the food preparation tips in the section "Putting the RAD Eating Plan into Action" on page 50.

WEIGHT-LOSS TRACK

Just three weeks to go until you've reached your ten-week, ten-pound target (that is, if you were following the plan to the letter and started your Weight-Loss Track in Week 3). Take some time this week to review your weekly records. If you've been able to lose a pound per week, then these records will serve as a guide for the rest of your journey. If you've lost somewhat less than this, you still have a road map to success. If you haven't lost any weight—or have even gained weight—then these records can serve as a starting point to discover what you can do differently. Are there areas where you can change your food choices? If so, what might you do? Was there a time when you seemed to reverse course? If there was, then why do you think it happened?

TIP FOR THE WEEK: *Beware using food to self-medicate stress.* Some fascinating animal and human studies (described in more detail on page 192) have affirmed what many people have known instinctively: When stress hits, it can often translate into an overwhelming desire for high-fat, sugary diet-busters. The reason, scientists have found, is that a high-fat, high-sugar diet actually works to calm the part of the brain that becomes overexcited in a stressful situation. For this reason, it's important to be extra aware of your eating habits when you're confronted with stress on the job or at home.

AEROBIC EXERCISE TRACK LEVELS I AND II

Level I exercisers, continue your current program. Level II exercisers, you have the option this week of staying at your current activity level or increasing your daily aerobic activity by another five minutes, to forty-five minutes per day, six days a week, with one rest day.

TIP FOR THE WEEK: *Breaking up your aerobic sessions.* Dividing your aerobic exercise sessions into shorter segments during the day can be a great way to fit in your aerobic exercise around a busy schedule. Evidence suggests that you'll get just as much benefit from aerobic exercise done in multiple sessions as short as ten minutes as you will from doing a fewer number of longer sessions—so long as you're still doing enough to hit the overall Diabetes Reset target of 150 minutes of moderate-intensity aerobic exercise per week.

STRENGTH TRAINING TRACK

Continue to do a full group of strength training exercises one or two days this week.

TIP FOR THE WEEK: *The lower-rep option.* I recommend doing ten to fifteen repetitions of each exercise because this number of repetitions allows you to increase the strength of your muscles using a moderate amount of resistance at a moderate intensity of effort. If you want to build strength and muscle mass more quickly, you can shift to a heavier resistance load—one that you are able to lift somewhere between eight and twelve times, with the last repetition feeling quite difficult. I advise doing this only if you are feeling extremely comfortable with your current ten-to-fifteen-repetition routine, however, and I also recommend checking with your doctor before shifting to this approach.

INFLAMMATION-FIGHTING TRACK

Continue to develop your inflammation-fighting strategy by seeking medical treatment for any chronic inflammatory conditions and adding anti-inflammatory foods and herbs to your daily menu.

TIP FOR THE WEEK: *Plants that heal.* The following herbs can help reduce inflammation throughout your body.

- *Turmeric/curcumin* has been found to lower CRP levels and reduce stiffness and swelling from rheumatoid arthritis, and may help counter early-stage Alzheimer's by inhibiting amyloid plaque formation. Products containing curcumin include Curamin (Terry Naturally, Europharma), a supplement product that also contains boswellia (another anti-inflammatory herb), and Meriva (Thorne Research, Now Foods, and Source Naturals).

- *Ginger* can reduce general inflammation, so drink fresh ginger tea and use fresh ginger for cooking. More powerful benefits can be gained from ginger extract capsules. Studies indicate ginger extract may help reduce arthritis-related knee inflammation and pain.

- *Zyflamend* is a supplement containing extracts of turmeric, ginger, rosemary, holy basil, Chinese knotweed, and other herbs.

- *Inflammatone* contains multiple anti-inflammatory herbs.

HEALTHY SLEEP TRACK

Continue taking steps to address any issues that are preventing you from getting seven to eight hours of restful sleep each night.

TIP FOR THE WEEK: *Sleep-promoting supplements.* The following natural supplements, all of which are available over the counter, may potentially improve sleep quality in some people. Because effects can vary among individuals, check with your doctor before trying any of these: melatonin (in capsule or sublingual lozenge form), chamomile tea, kava kava tea, valerian, gamma-aminobutyric acid (GABA), 5-hydroxytryptophan (5-HTP), and tryptophan (which not only boosts levels of the sleep-enhancing neurotransmitter serotonin but also appears to stimulate the growth of new insulin-producing beta cells in the pancreas, according to new research).

ANTI-STRESS TRACK

This week, continue to focus on your stress management strategies. At the end of the week, write down which strategies seem to be working best in a notebook or journal.

TIP FOR THE WEEK: *The magic of meditation.* Numerous studies have shown that meditative breathing is one of the most effective ways to defuse your "fight of flight" nervous response—the increased breathing and heart rate and other physiological changes triggered by stress. It's done by closing your eyes, relaxing, then inhaling and exhaling slowly through your nose for several minutes or longer as you silently repeat a single calm-inducing word, sound, or short phrase with each in-breath and out-breath, keeping your thoughts focused on this word, sound, or phrase throughout.

NATURAL ANTIOXIDANTS TRACK

Continue to incorporate plants and herbs that are rich in Phase 2 antioxidants into your daily RAD eating plan.

TIP FOR THE WEEK: *Add herbal supplements for extra antioxidant effects.* Consider expanding your antioxidant strategy by adding concentrated herbal sources of Phase 2 antioxidants to your daily eating plan. These include broccoli seed extract, curcumin or turmeric extract, milk thistle, bacopa extract, and ashwagandha root powder.

Diabetes Reset Calendar—Week 10

DAY 1

Daily aerobic activity (minutes) _____

Strength workout (yes/no) _____

Hours slept _____

Daily food totals

Total grams fiber _____

Total grams fat _____

Total calories _____

Target calories _____

Current weight _____

DAY 2

Daily aerobic activity (minutes) _____

Strength workout (yes/no) _____

Hours slept _____

Daily food totals

Total grams fiber _____

Total grams fat _____

Total calories _____

Target calories _____

Current weight _____

DAY 3

Daily aerobic activity (minutes) _____

Strength workout (yes/no) _____

Hours slept _____

Daily food totals

Total grams fiber _____

Total grams fat _____

Total calories _____

Target calories _____

Current weight _____

DAY 4

Daily aerobic activity (minutes) _____

Strength workout (yes/no) _____

Hours slept _____

Daily food totals

Total grams fiber _____

Total grams fat _____

Total calories _____

Target calories _____

Current weight _____

DAY 5

Daily aerobic activity (minutes) _____

Strength workout (yes/no) _____

Hours slept _____

Daily food totals

Total grams fiber _____

Total grams fat _____

Total calories _____

Target calories _____

Current weight _____

DAY 6

Daily aerobic activity (minutes) ____

Strength workout (yes/no) _____

Hours slept _____

Daily food totals

Total grams fiber _____

Total grams fat _____

Total calories _____

Target calories _____

Current weight _____

DAY 7

Daily aerobic activity (minutes) ____

Strength workout (yes/no) _____

Hours slept _____

Daily food totals

Total grams fiber _____

Total grams fat _____

Total calories _____

Target calories _____

Starting weight _____

Goal weight _____

Current weight _____

Pounds lost _____

Week 11: Optimizing Your Vitamin D

GOALS FOR THE WEEK

- Continue maintaining your RAD eating plan and, if necessary, your weight-loss plan.

- Aerobic Exercise Track Level I: Continue your walking program of 2,500 steps/twenty-five minutes of brisk walking per day, with one rest day per week.

- Aerobic Exercise Track Level II: Either maintain your current activity level or add five additional minutes per day for a daily total of forty-five minutes of brisk walking or other moderate-intensity aerobic exercise, with one rest day per week.

- Continue your strength training program of two resistance exercise sessions per week.

- Continue your anti-inflammation, healthy sleeping, stress management, natural antioxidant, and brown fat-activation strategies.

- This week, as the final piece of your Diabetes Reset strategy, review your Vitamin D levels and consider taking supplements if necessary.

Week 11: Overview

NEW: VITAMIN D TRACK

A majority of Americans in the northern section of the country have been found to suffer at least part of the time from vitamin D deficiencies, which in turn has been linked to increased risk for metabolic syndrome and type 2 diabetes. This week, I encourage you to have your vitamin D levels checked—many primary care and family physicians now order this test routinely as part of their patients' annual exams, and you can also request a lab test on your own.

TIP FOR THE WEEK: *Treating low vitamin D levels.* If your vitamin D levels are less than optimal, consult with your doctor about taking vitamin D supplements. Both vitamin D3 and D2 have been found effective, but D3 has been shown to be somewhat superior over the longer term. Vitamin D deficiency is typically corrected first with a loading regimen of prescription-strength vitamin D—50,000 IU taken orally, either once weekly for several months or several times weekly for one month. Once vitamin D has reached normal levels, daily over-the-counter supplements of 800 IU to 1,000 IU vitamin D3 should be sufficient to maintain these levels.

HEALTHY EATING TRACK

Continue to implement the RAD eating plan while tracking your daily fiber and fat consumption.

TIP FOR THE WEEK: *Look to legumes.* Rich in micronutrients, exceptionally high in fiber, tasty, and filling, legumes are a multitasker. With more than 7 grams of fiber per half cup, lentils and black beans are powerhouse menu choices for lunch or dinner—and lima beans, kidney beans, and chickpeas, at more than 6 grams of fiber per half cup, aren't far behind, with chickpea-based hummus weighing in at more than 7 grams of fiber per half cup.

WEIGHT-LOSS TRACK

In this, the next-to-last week of your ten-week program, take some time to compliment yourself on everything you've done right, whether or not you've managed to achieve your one pound per week weight-loss goal. You are eating better, leading a more physically active life, and have taken steps not only to lose body fat but also to improve many other aspects of your health and well-being. Whatever weight you may be now, you are fashioning a path to better future health, and for that I congratulate you.

TIP FOR THE WEEK: *Practice mindful eating.* Key elements of this approach include eating only when you actually feel hungry, selecting a calm, pleasant setting for meals, and avoiding looking at your smartphone or multitasking when sitting down to eat. Instead, focus your attention on the taste, smell, and texture of your food, both on the plate and as you're chewing and swallowing it. Mindful eating also stresses chewing each mouthful at least ten times, taking time to converse and sip from your water glass between bites, and being willing to leave food uneaten on your plate once you reach a point where you feel full.

AEROBIC EXERCISE TRACK LEVELS I AND II

Level I exercisers, continue your current program. Level II exercisers, you have the option this week of staying at your current activity level or increasing your daily aerobic activity by another five minutes, to fifty minutes per day, six days a week, with one rest day.

TIP FOR THE WEEK: *Speedplay.* As your endurance and stamina improve, one way to continue enhancing your fitness without spending more time on your actual workout is to add some stretches of increased effort during the course of each walk, bicycle ride, run, or swimming session. This could mean increasing your pace for one minute and then slow back down to your original pace (or even slower for a stretch of time, if needed to recover from the effort). Or you could pick an object in the near distance—a particular landmark—and decide to walk, run, or cycle at a slightly faster clip until you reach that destination. In addition to boosting your cardiovascular fitness, there is also evidence that increasing the intensity of your aerobic exercise can further increase insulin sensitivity.

STRENGTH TRAINING TRACK

Continue to do a full group of strength training exercises one or two days this week.

INFLAMMATION-FIGHTING TRACK

Continue to develop your inflammation-fighting strategy by seeking medical treatment for any chronic inflammatory conditions and adding anti-inflammatory foods and herbs to your daily menu.

TIP FOR THE WEEK: *Avoiding air pollution.* Smog and car exhaust contribute to inflammation, insulin resistance, and type 2 diabetes risk. To minimize your exposure, avoid exercising outdoors in smoggy conditions or in areas with heavy automobile traffic and consider buying a HEPA filter or electrostatic air filter for your home.

HEALTHY SLEEP TRACK

Continue taking steps to address any issues that are preventing you from getting seven to eight hours of restful sleep each night.

TIP FOR THE WEEK: *Treating sleep apnea.* If you snore at night or have frequent breathing stoppages when you're sleeping, then you may be suffering from sleep apnea—a sleep disorder in which your throat collapses shut repeatedly during the night, blocking your airway. In addition to impairing sleep quality and leading to daytime drowsiness, sleep apnea has been linked to significantly increased risk for type 2 diabetes as well as other conditions. If you think you may have it, discuss treatment options with your doctor, including the possibility of getting a CPAP (continuous positive airway pressure) machine (see page 179).

ANTI-STRESS TRACK

This week, continue to focus on your stress management strategies. At the end of the week, write down which strategies seem to be working best in the Notes section of your weekly calendar.

TIP FOR THE WEEK: *Consider counseling.* For ongoing chronic stress, stress-reduction exercises often aren't enough. Psychotherapy, and cognitive-behavioral therapy in particular, has been shown to be one of the most effective ways to relieve persistent anxiety and other stress-related symptoms.

NATURAL ANTIOXIDANTS TRACK

Continue to incorporate plants and herbs that are rich in Phase 2 anti-oxidants into your daily RAD eating plan.

TIP FOR THE WEEK: *Super supplements.* To maximize your body's antioxidant defenses, you may also want to consider trying Nrf2 Activate, manufactured by Health Naturally. This supplement, developed by a physician, contains a number of herbs known to stimulate the body's Nrf2 pathways: sulfurophane, curcumin, pterostilbene, green tea extract, and black pepper extract.

BROWN FAT ACTIVATION TRACK

Continue to explore ways to activate your brown fat stores, both during your normal daily routine and during your exercise sessions.

DIABETES RESET CALENDAR—WEEK 11

DAY 1

Daily aerobic activity (minutes) _____

Strength workout (yes/no) _____

Hours slept _____

Daily food totals

Total grams fiber _____

Total grams fat _____

Total calories _____

Target calories _____

Current weight _____

DAY 2

Daily aerobic activity (minutes) _____

Strength workout (yes/no) _____

Hours slept _____

Daily food totals

Total grams fiber _____

Total grams fat _____

Total calories _____

Target calories _____

Current weight _____

DAY 3

Daily aerobic activity (minutes) _____

Strength workout (yes/no) _____

Hours slept _____

Daily food totals

Total grams fiber _____

Total grams fat _____

Total calories _____

Target calories _____

Current weight _____

DAY 4

Daily aerobic activity (minutes) _____

Strength workout (yes/no) _____

Hours slept _____

Daily food totals

Total grams fiber _____

Total grams fat _____

Total calories _____

Target calories _____

Current weight _____

DAY 5

Daily aerobic activity (minutes) _____

Strength workout (yes/no) _____

Hours slept _____

Daily food totals

Total grams fiber _____

Total grams fat _____

Total calories _____

Target calories _____

Current weight _____

DAY 6

Daily aerobic activity (minutes) _____

Strength workout (yes/no) _____

Hours slept _____

Daily food totals

Total grams fiber _____

Total grams fat _____

Total calories _____

Target calories _____

Current weight _____

DAY 7

Daily aerobic activity (minutes) ____	**Daily food totals**
Strength workout (yes/no) _____	Total grams fiber _____
Hours slept _____	Total grams fat _____
	Total calories _____
	Target calories _____
	Starting weight _____
	Current weight _____
	Pounds lost _____
	Goal weight _____

Week 12: The Diabetes Reset Lifetime Plan

GOALS FOR THE WEEK

- Maintain all strategy tracks for the week.

- Complete your ten-week weight-loss program and record your weight loss.

- Develop a plan for carrying your Diabetes Reset strategies forward in a way that can be sustained permanently.

Week 12: Overview

NEW: CONGRATULATIONS!

You have successfully implemented all of the Diabetes Reset strategies for improving your insulin sensitivity, protecting the insulin-producing cells of your pancreas, and enhancing your body's ability to metabolize blood glucose. Your challenge now is to continue the Diabetes Reset Plan in the years ahead. In this week's notes following, I'll discuss how best to do this. Meanwhile, I urge you to keep a record as you progress on your own journey of health—in a private journal, a blog, a personal calendar—and also to share what you have done and are continuing to do with others, so that they can benefit from this approach as well.

GLUCOSE CHECK 3

During this week, pick two days and use a blood glucose home test kit to do a final check of your blood glucose levels. As before, check your blood glucose four times on each of those days—when you first wake up, and then again one hour after each meal—then compare these sets of readings and their average to your other two sets of glucose readings. If you have implemented all of the relevant Diabetes Reset strategies, your average readings should be significantly lower than they were at the start of the Twelve-Week Diabetes Reset Plan.

HEALTHY EATING TRACK

You have adopted an approach to eating that will help protect and enhance your health for the rest of your life. Here is my challenge to you for the future: Write down what the most successful and least successful elements of your Healthy Eating Track have been—what aspects were fun and easy, as well as what you found difficult or confusing. Then write down a set of personal guidelines that will help you maintain the RAD eating plan in the months and years ahead—a list that could include your favorite meal plans and recipes, too.

WEIGHT-LOSS TRACK

Congratulations on sticking to your ten-week plan. If you have lost 5% to 7% of your starting weight or have reached a BMI of less than 25, then I recommend shifting to the normal RAD eating plan, without caloric restriction. If you need to lose a bit more to reach at least a 5% weight loss, then continue on the Diabetes Reset Weight-Loss Track until you do. In addition, if your BMI is still over 25 and you want to continue on this track until you reach that goal, do it!

AEROBIC EXERCISE TRACK LEVELS I AND II

Hats off to both Level I and Level II exercisers: You have achieved one of the most critical goals in your Diabetes Reset Plan. Your challenge now is to develop a plan that will enable you to maintain this level of aerobic activity in the future. Continue to schedule daily aerobic sessions and be on guard for any obstacles that block you from this essential task. From time to time, you may want to go back and reread Strategy Chapter 3 to remind yourself of what a valuable gift these twenty-five minutes (or more) of daily physical activity really are.

STRENGTH TRAINING TRACK

Like aerobic exercise, regular strength training is one of the best ways available to increase your insulin sensitivity and prevent the occurrence or progression of type 2 diabetes. As with the Aerobic Exercise Track, I challenge you now to develop a plan that will enable you to maintain your strength training program over the months and years ahead.

INFLAMMATION-FIGHTING TRACK

Fighting inflammation is a lifelong process. As you continue to implement the inflammation-fighting strategies in this book, I recommend engaging in an ongoing dialogue with your doctor about addressing any inflammation or infection that arises in the future.

HEALTHY SLEEP TRACK

As Strategy Chapter 6 of this book makes clear, getting a consistently good night's sleep is one of the most important things you can do for your glucose metabolism and overall health. I strongly recommend that you continue to aggressively implement the prosleep strategies outlined in *The Diabetes Reset* and that you also seek out a sleep specialist if you experience ongoing issues regarding your sleep quality or quantity.

ANTI-STRESS TRACK

Stress is an often inescapable part of life. I hope, however, that this book has convinced you to take a serious approach toward managing any chronic stress you are experiencing and also to aggressively seek treatment from an experienced psychiatrist, psychologist, or therapist for any depression or anxiety that may be affecting you.

NATURAL ANTIOXIDANTS TRACK

The power of Phase 2 antioxidants to unleash your body's natural protective substances is quite remarkable. In the months and years ahead, I hope you will reread Strategy Chapter 8 on occasion and continue to employ the tips outlined there.

BROWN FAT ACTIVATION TRACK

Your body's stores of this unique fat are a "secret weapon" for maintaining a healthy weight. In the months and years ahead, continue to review Strategy Chapter 4 from time to time—and remember that a sub-70° F environment is the key to activating brown fat's significant calorie-burning potential.

VITAMIN D TRACK

Optimal vitamin D levels are essential for optimal health. Continue to monitor your vitamin D levels in the years ahead, getting prescription supplementation if you're deficient and taking 800 IU to 1,000 IU per day of vitamin D3 supplements to maintain healthy levels.

DIABETES RESET CALENDAR—WEEK 12
LIFETIME PROGRAM

DAY 1

Daily aerobic activity (minutes)
_____

Strength workout (yes/no) _____

Hours slept _____

Daily food totals

Total grams fiber _____

Total grams fat _____

Total calories _____

Target calories _____

Current weight _____

DAY 2

Daily aerobic activity (minutes)

_____

Strength workout (yes/no) _____

Hours slept _____

Daily food totals

Total grams fiber _____

Total grams fat _____

Total calories _____

Target calories _____

Current weight _____

DAY 3

Daily aerobic activity (minutes)

_____

Strength workout (yes/no) _____

Hours slept _____

Daily food totals

Total grams fiber _____

Total grams fat _____

Total calories _____

Target calories _____

Current weight _____

DAY 4

Daily aerobic activity (minutes)

_____

Strength workout (yes/no) _____

Hours slept _____

Daily food totals

Total grams fiber _____

Total grams fat _____

Total calories _____

Target calories _____

Current weight _____

DAY 5

Daily aerobic activity (minutes)

_____

Strength workout (yes/no) _____

Hours slept _____

Daily food totals

Total grams fiber _____

Total grams fat _____

Total calories _____

Target calories _____

Current weight _____

DAY 6

Daily aerobic activity (minutes)

_____

Strength workout (yes/no) _____

Hours slept _____

Daily food totals

Total grams fiber _____

Total grams fat _____

Total calories _____

Target calories _____

Current weight _____

DAY 7

Daily aerobic activity (minutes)

_____

Strength workout (yes/no) _____

Hours slept _____

Daily food totals

Total grams fiber _____

Total grams fat _____

Total calories _____

Target calories _____

Current weight _____

Goal weight _____

Start weight _____

Ten-week weight loss _____

STRATEGIES TO PREVENT OR CONTROL GESTATIONAL DIABETES

The insulin-enhancing strategies outlined in this book are vitally important for another populous group that I've mentioned only in passing up until now: women who have been or are currently pregnant, or who might become pregnant in the foreseeable future. This is because pregnancy causes expecting mothers to become *highly insulin resistant,* particularly during their third trimester. The dramatic jump in insulin resistance during pregnancy arises mainly from the various hormones released by the placenta, which interfere with insulin's action in the mother's skeletal muscles and fat tissues. Excessive body fat gained during pregnancy can contribute to pregnancy-related insulin resistance as well, for the same reasons that obesity contributes to diabetes risk in those who aren't pregnant.

As the fetus grows larger, this insulin-blunting effect becomes so strong that it can reduce the mother's insulin sensitivity by 50%. As a result, pregnant women must produce substantially more insulin than usual in order to transport glucose from their blood into their muscles, fat tissue, and other insulin-dependent organs. In fact, the amount of insulin manufactured by a pregnant woman's pancreas typically doubles or triples in her third trimester. Although the majority of women produce enough insulin to keep their blood glucose levels within a normal range, a certain percentage of women are unable to manufacture enough insulin to overcome this pregnancy-related insulin resistance. As a result, their blood glucose levels become elevated, a condition known as *gestational diabetes.* If this occurs, then the mother will need to control her glucose levels by taking medication—usually insulin—for the duration of her pregnancy in order to protect her unborn child from the ill effects of elevated blood glucose.

The Health Risks of Gestational Diabetes

G estational diabetes poses health risks for both the mother and child. The danger for the mother is both short and long term: The short-term risk for the mother is an increase in complications during pregnancy and delivery, including elevated risk of preeclampsia (a dangerous condition that causes high blood pressure and can damage the kidneys and other organs) and the various problems associated with delivering a large baby (as discussed next). The longer-term issue is that women who develop gestational diabetes have a significantly heightened risk of developing type 2 diabetes later in life. The latest data indicate that a woman who has been diagnosed with gestational diabetes has a 50% chance of getting type 2 diabetes within seven to ten years after delivering her baby. Having gestational diabetes also increases the risk that you will develop the same condition in subsequent pregnancies.

The main risks for the baby occur during the pregnancy and immediately afterward. For women who already have diabetes at the start of pregnancy, elevated blood glucose levels early in pregnancy can cause birth defects or even miscarriage, which is why pregnant type 1 women are monitored extremely closely. For the offspring of women who are not diabetic prior to becoming pregnant but who go on to develop gestational diabetes, the risk lies in the later months of pregnancy. Because the mother's insulin cannot cross the placenta, the baby must produce extra insulin to manage his or her elevated glucose levels. While this response keeps the baby's blood glucose normalized, all that extra glucose that the baby is now metabolizing has to go somewhere—and so it is converted into fat, causing the baby to grow larger than normal. In addition, insulin has growth-promoting effects, which may also contribute to the size of the fetus.

This "big baby" effect can make delivery more dangerous, and may also put the child at greater risk of being overweight and developing type 2 diabetes later in life. The baby's elevated insulin levels can also cause a dangerous drop in blood glucose and related respiratory distress immediately after delivery, when the baby is abruptly deprived of the mother's blood glucose supply.

Getting Tested for Gestational Diabetes

Pregnant women will typically be tested for gestational diabetes around the twenty-fourth week of pregnancy. Testing may take place earlier in pregnancy if a urine sample shows abnormally high glucose levels, or if a woman is considered at high risk of gestational diabetes due to a BMI of 30 or higher, a previous diagnosis of gestational diabetes, or a family history of diabetes.

With new research indicating that babies can show effects of gestational diabetes at lower maternal blood glucose levels than previously thought, the approach to glucose testing for pregnant women is shifting as well.

Traditional testing method
Traditionally, testing for gestational diabetes has involved a two-part process. First, all women would undergo a glucose-screening test, in which they drink a liquid containing 50 grams of glucose, then have their blood drawn 60 minutes later to check their blood glucose level. If this level is more than 130 mg/dL, the woman then returns on another day for a three-hour fasting oral glucose tolerance test, in which she fasts for at least eight hours, then drinks a liquid

containing 100 grams of glucose. Four blood measurements are taken during the test—one just before drinking the liquid, then additional draws one hour, two hours, and three hours after ingesting the glucose. If two out of four readings are elevated, it's considered an indication of gestational diabetes.

Proposed new testing method
Under the new, more rigorous criteria for gestational diabetes that have been proposed, all pregnant women would be given a two-hour fasting oral glucose tolerance test in which three blood readings are taken: a fasting measurement, followed by measurements at one and two hours after ingesting a dose of glucose. A diagnosis of gestational diabetes is made if one out of the three readings is elevated.

At Joslin, we are currently following the newer testing guidelines. The medical community as a whole continues to be divided over which approach to follow, however. If you are pregnant, I recommend that you discuss these different testing approaches with your doctor and come to a mutual decision on how to proceed.

Why Gestational Diabetes May Be More Common Than Previously Believed

Until recently, it was estimated that 3.5% of pregnant European American and African American women develop gestational diabetes, with higher rates for Hispanic American women (6%), East Asian American women (8%), and South Asian American women (11%). These rates were based on blood glucose readings during pregnancy that had been linked to increased risk of type 2 diabetes in later life.

Over the past several years, however, rigorous studies have found that babies are at risk of having elevated insulin levels and becoming abnormally large even when the mother's blood glucose is elevated only slightly—to levels that previously would not have resulted in their being diagnosed and treated for gestational diabetes (See box on page 307: Getting Tested for Gestational Diabetes.) As these new guidelines get incorporated into physicians' practices, the expectation is that a greater percentage of women will end up being treated for gestational diabetes in the years to come.

Using the Diabetes Reset Strategies to Prevent and Manage Gestational Diabetes

B ecause all of the Diabetes Reset strategies are designed to enhance your body's insulin sensitivity and protect the ability of your pancreas to produce insulin, they all have value in helping your body meet the heightened insulin demand that occurs during pregnancy. In particular, the first three Diabetes Reset strategies—the Rural Asian Diet, weight loss, and increased physical activity—appear to benefit women before, during, and after pregnancy.

PREPARING FOR PREGNANCY

Using these strategies to optimize your glucose metabolism *before* you become pregnant will give you the best chances of avoiding this condition. Research has shown that women who develop gestational diabetes typically have signs of impaired glucose metabolism before pregnancy, and that the stress of pregnancy itself causes these impairments to become evident.

One of the most important things you can do to prepare for pregnancy is to follow the high-fiber, low-fat RAD eating plan outlined in

Strategy Chapter 1. Avoiding animal fat and dietary cholesterol (found primarily in organ meats and shellfish) appears to be particularly important: In a groundbreaking 2012 study by researchers at the National Institutes of Health (NIH) and Harvard that drew from data on 13,000 women compiled in the Nurses' Health Study II, women who ate the most animal fat in the years prior to pregnancy were twice as likely to develop gestational diabetes as those who consumed the least animal fat, while those who consumed the most cholesterol were 45% more likely to be diagnosed than those with the lowest cholesterol intake.

Maintaining a healthy weight prior to becoming pregnant is also important. While the extent of the association remains uncertain, being overweight at the onset of pregnancy has been found to substantially increase risk of developing gestational diabetes. Finally, getting regular exercise in the years before you become pregnant is another key factor. A meta-analysis led by Harvard researchers found that the women who were most active prior to pregnancy had 55% less risk of developing gestational diabetes than those who were least active.

DURING PREGNANCY

Your doctor is the best source of advice in terms of nutrition and physical exercise during pregnancy. That being said, there is good evidence that gaining excessive weight while pregnant, especially early in pregnancy, increases the risk of gestational diabetes. Conversely, exercise appears to play a protective role early in pregnancy. The Harvard meta-analysis that looked at benefits of pre-pregnancy exercise also found that study subjects who were most active in the first months of their pregnancy reduced their risk of gestational diabetes by about 25%, compared to the least active subjects.

For these reasons, I recommend you discuss with your doctor the benefits of a high-fiber diet rich in complex carbohydrates as well as regular, moderate physical exercise during pregnancy. You should also pay close attention to any sleep problems you may be experiencing. In one study, women with gestational diabetes were seven times more likely to be suffering from sleep apnea.

AFTER PREGNANCY

For women who have been diagnosed with gestational diabetes, taking aggressive steps to address your diabetes risk factors following your pregnancy should be a top priority. Exercise appears to be an especially critical factor in reducing your long-term risk of developing type 2 diabetes. A recently published NIH study analyzed data compiled by the Nurses' Health Study II on more than 4,500 women who were previously diagnosed with gestational diabetes. It found that those who got at least 150 minutes of moderate physical activity each week—the same amount recommended by the Diabetes Reset exercise strategy—reduced their risk of eventually developing type 2 diabetes by 47%, compared to those who were least active. I should add that this protective effect was found to occur *regardless* of the subjects' body weight.

The bottom line: If you are currently pregnant or envision becoming pregnant one day—or if you were diagnosed with gestational diabetes at some point during a pregnancy—then the various diabetes-fighting strategies outlined in *The Diabetes Reset* offer powerful benefits for your own health, and that of your children.

ENDNOTES

INTRODUCTION

80% of people with type 2 diabetes are overweight or obese: National Institute of Diabetes and Digestive and Kidney Diseases (NIDDK), National Diabetes Information Clearinghouse. *Diabetes Overview.* diabetes.niddk.nih.gov/dm/pubs/overview/.

STRATEGY CHAPTER 1

every one of them showed significant improvement in their insulin sensitivity: Hsu, W., et al. "Improvement of insulin sensitivity by isoenergy high carbohydrate traditional Asian diet: a randomized controlled pilot feasibility study." *PLOS ONE* 9 (2014): e106851.

Two thirds of adult Americans are now overweight or obese: Flegal, K. M., et al. "Prevalence of Obesity and Trends in the Distribution of Body Mass Index Among U.S. Adults, 1999–2010." *JAMA* 307 (2012): 491–497.

at least 26 million Americans have type 2 diabetes, and another 86 million have prediabetes: Centers for Disease Control and Prevention. *National Diabetes Statistics Report, 2014.* cdc.gov/diabetes/pubs/statsreport14.htm.

if you look at USDA data on Americans' food intake from 1970 to 2010: U.S. Department of Agriculture. *Food Availability (Per Capita) Data System: Summary Findings.* http://ers.usda.gov/data-products/food-availability-(per-capita)-data -system/summary-findings.

the amount of physical activity Americans get each day actually declined: Brownson, R. C., et al. "Declining rates of physical activity in the United States: what are the contributors?" *Annu Rev Public Health* 26 (2005): 421–443.

In a number of studies of mice who were genetically altered: Cohen, S. E., et al. "High circulating leptin receptors with normal leptin sensitivity in liver-specific insulin receptor knock-out (LIRKO) mice." *J Biol Chem* 282 (2007): 23672–23678.

grams of daily fat consumed by the average American remained virtually unchanged: Centers for Disease Control and Prevention. "Trends in Intake of Energy and Macronutrients—United States, 1971–2000." *MMWR* 53 (2004): 80–82.

Because human beings' protein intake tends to remain remarkably constant: Fulgoni, V. L. "Current protein intake in America: analysis of the National Health and Nutrition Examination Survey, 2003–2004." *Am J Clin Nutr* 87 (2008):1554S–1557S.

the percentage of Chinese with diabetes now stands at 11.6%: Xu, Y., et al. "Prevalence and control of diabetes in Chinese adults." *JAMA* 310 (2013): 948–959.

When obesity-resistant rats were fed a high-fat diet during pregnancy: Strakovsky, R. S., et al. "Gestational high fat diet programs hepatic phosphoenolpyruvate carboxykinase gene expression and histone modification in neonatal offspring rats." *J Physiol* 589 (2011): 2707–2717.

A recent report showed that changing from a vegetarian diet: David, L. A., et al. "Diet rapidly and reproducibly alters the human gut microbiome." *Nature* 505 (2014): 559–563.

high-fiber diets have been associated with reduced blood levels of C-reactive protein: Neuhouser, M. L., et al. "A low-glycemic load diet reduces serum C-reactive protein and modestly increases adiponectin in overweight and obese adults." *J Nutr* 142 (2012): 369–374.

short-chain fatty acids that fiber produces when it ferments in the intestinal tract: Robertson, M. D., et al. "Insulin-sensitizing effects of dietary resistant starch and effects on skeletal muscle and adipose tissue metabolism." *Am J Clin Nutr* 82 (2005): 559–567.

intestinal fermentation of fiber—particularly insoluble fiber—has been shown to stimulate production of glucose: De Vadder, F., et al. "Microbiota-generated metabolites promote metabolic benefits via gut-brain neural circuits." *Cell* 156 (2014): 84–96.

People who are overweight or obese appear to have chronically higher FFA levels: Jensen, M. D., et al. "Influence of body fat distribution on free fatty acid metabolism in obesity." *J Clin Invest* 83 (1989): 1168–1173.

elevated FFA levels in the blood can cause signs of insulin resistance within two to four hours: Boden, G. "Effects of free fatty acids (FFA) on glucose metabolism: significance for insulin resistance and type 2 diabetes." *Exp Clin Endocrinol Diabetes* 111 (2003): 121–124.

studies have also found that suppressing FFA levels for just twelve hours: Santomauro, A. T., et al. "Overnight lowering of free fatty acids with Acipimox improves insulin resistance and glucose tolerance in obese diabetic and nondiabetic subjects." *Diabetes* 48 (1999): 1836-1841.

the same fermentation process that signals the body to become more responsive to insulin: Weickert, M.O., et al. "Metabolic effects of dietary fiber consumption and prevention of diabetes." *J Nutr* 138 (2008): 439–442.

people who eat diets high in fiber feel more "full" after eating: Clark, M. J., et al. "The effect of fiber on satiety and food intake: a systematic review." *J Am Coll Nutr* 32 (2013): 200–211.

the more fiber people eat, the lower their body weight and body fat tends to be: Slavin, J. L. "Dietary fiber and body weight." *Nutrition* 21 (2005): 411–418.

The Finnish Diabetes Prevention Study made history: Lindström, J., et al. "The Finnish Diabetes Prevention Study (DPS): Lifestyle intervention and 3-year results on diet and physical activity." *Diabetes Care* 26 (2003): 3230–3236.

An even larger U.S. study, the Diabetes Prevention Program: Knowler, W. C., et al. "Reduction in the incidence of type 2 diabetes with lifestyle intervention or metformin." *N Engl J Med* 346 (2002): 393–403.

a study published in 2011 by our colleagues at the Harvard University School of Public Health: Pan, A., et al. "Red meat consumption and risk of type 2 diabetes: 3 cohorts of US adults and an updated meta-analysis." *Am J Clin Nutr* 94 (2011): 1088–1096.

STRATEGY CHAPTER 2

In 2009, a team of Canadian researchers published a meta-analysis: Guh, D. P., et al. "The incidence of co-morbidities related to obesity and overweight: A systematic review and meta-analysis." *BMC Public Health* 9 (2009): 88.

men and women in this category are about forty times more likely to develop type 2 diabetes: Chan, J. M., et al. "Obesity, fat distribution, and weight gain as risk factors for clinical diabetes in men." *Diabetes Care* 17 (1994): 961–969.
Shai, I., et al. "Ethnicity, Obesity, and Risk of Type 2 Diabetes in Women—A 20-year follow-up study." *Diabetes Care* 29 (2006): 1585–1590.

36% of American adults—slightly more than one third—are obese: Flegal, K. M., et al. "Prevalence of Obesity and Trends in the Distribution of Body Mass Index Among US Adults, 1999–2010." *JAMA* 307 (2012): 491–497.

between 8% and 9% of the adult population in the United States has type 2 diabetes: Centers for Disease Control and Prevention. *National Diabetes Statistics Report, 2014.* cdc.gov/diabetes/pubs/statsreport14.htm.

Studies suggest that one reason for this somewhat protective effect: Barbarroja, N., et al. "The obese healthy paradox: is inflammation the answer?" *Biochem J* 15 (2010): 141–149.

lean individuals, particularly those with two parents who were diagnosed with type 2 diabetes: Petersen K. F., et al. "Impaired mitochondrial activity in the insulin-resistant offspring of patients with type 2 diabetes." *N Engl J Med* 350 (2004): 664–671.

Proteins that appear to play a role in this process include: Kershaw, E. E., et al. "Adipose Tissue as an Endocrine Organ." *J Clin Endocrinol Metab* 89 (2004): 2548–2556.

Joslin scientists reported on a pivotal study linking insulin resistance: Cai, D., et al. "Local and systemic insulin resistance resulting from hepatic activation of IKK-beta and NF-kappaB." *Nat Med* 11 (2005): 183–190.

A 2011 study published in the Journal of Clinical Endocrinology & Metabolism: Sung, K.-C., et al. "Interrelationship between fatty liver and insulin resistance in the development of type 2 diabetes." *J Clin Endocrinol Metab* 96 (2011): 1093–1097.

In 2012, the CDC released a study projecting that if current trends hold: Finkelstein, E. A., et al. "Obesity and Severe Obesity Forecasts Through 2030." *Am J Prev Med* 42 (2012): 563–570.

The Diabetes Prevention Program (DPP) was a federally funded, multicenter study: Knowler, W. C., et al. "Reduction in the incidence of type 2 diabetes with lifestyle intervention or metformin." *N Engl J Med* 346 (2002): 393–403.

The Look AHEAD Study was launched in 2001: Look AHEAD Research Group. "Long-term effects of a lifestyle intervention on weight and cardiovascular risk factors in individuals with type 2 diabetes mellitus: four-year results of the Look AHEAD trial." *Arch Intern Med* 170 (2010): 1566–1575.

In 2008, Joslin published a study of five different groups: Hamdy, O., et al. "Why WAIT Program: A Novel Model for Diabetes Weight Management in Routine Clinical Practice." *Obesity Management* 4 (2008): 176–183.

In a nationwide study that looked at changes in food consumption patterns from 1977 to 1998: Nielsen, S. J., et al. "Patterns and trends in food portion sizes, 1977–1998." *JAMA* 289 (2003): 450–453.

a 2007 study analyzing three thousand members of the National Weight Control Registry: Butryn, M. L., et al. "Consistent self-monitoring of weight: a key component of successful weight loss maintenance." *Obesity* 15 (2007): 3091–3096.

In a groundbreaking clinical trial at the Cleveland Clinic: Schauer, P. R., et al. "Bariatric surgery versus intensive medical therapy in obese patients with diabetes." *N Engl J Med* 366 (2012): 1567–1576.

STRATEGY CHAPTER 3

The seven-minute workout that has gotten media attention: Klika, B., et al. "High-intensity circuit training using body weight: maximum results with minimal investment." *ACSM's Health & Fitness Journal* 17 (2013): 8–13.

A meta-analysis of fourteen studies of exercise interventions: Thomas, D. E., et al. "Exercise for type 2 diabetes mellitus." *Cochrane Database Syst Rev* 19 (2006): CD002968.

well-known study that followed six thousand male University of Pennsylvania graduates: Helmrich, S. P., et al. "Physical activity and reduced occurrence of non-insulin-dependent diabetes mellitus." *N Engl J Med* 325 (1991): 147–152.

In one controlled study that compared diet and exercise to dieting alone: Tamura, Y., et al. "Effects of diet and exercise on muscle and liver intracellular lipid contents and insulin sensitivity in type 2 diabetic patients." *J Clin Endocrinol Metab* 90 (2005): 3191–3196.

A review of thirteen randomized controlled trials that was published in 2010: Strasser, B., et al. "Resistance training in the treatment of the metabolic syndrome: a systematic review and meta-analysis of the effect of resistance training on metabolic clustering in patients with abnormal glucose metabolism." *Sports Med* 40 (2010): 397–415.

An analysis of thirteen thousand adult subjects: Srikanthan, P., et al. "Relative muscle mass is inversely associated with insulin resistance and prediabetes. Findings from the third National Health and Nutrition Examination Survey." *J Clin Endocrinol Metab* 96 (2011): 2898–2903.

STRATEGY CHAPTER 4

Several years ago, Dr. Cypess teamed up with other Joslin colleagues: Cypess, A. M., et al. "Identification and importance of brown adipose tissue in adult humans." *N Engl J Med* 360 (2009): 1509–1517.

investigators in the Netherlands scanned twenty-four men: van Marken Lichtenbelt, W. D., et al. "Cold-activated brown adipose tissue in healthy men." *N Engl J Med* 360 (2009): 1500–1508.

In another study, Swedish researchers scanned five subjects: Virtanen, K. A., et al. "Functional brown adipose tissue in healthy adults." *N Engl J Med* 360 (2009): 1518–1525.

experiments have shown that within just five minutes of donning the vests: Cypess, A. M., et al. "Cold but not sympathomimetics activates human brown adipose tissue in vivo." *Proc Natl Acad Sci USA* 109 (2012): 10001–1005.

One group of investigators, for example, recently found that a certain protein: Müller, T. D., et al. "p62 Links β-adrenergic input to mitochondrial function and thermogenesis." *J Clin Invest* 123 (2013): 469–478.

In another research project, conducted here at Joslin in Dr. Laurie Goodyear's section: Stanford, K. I., et al. "Brown adipose tissue regulates glucose homeostasis and insulin sensitivity." *J Clin Invest* 123 (2013): 215–223.

scientists at Joslin led by Dr. Yu-Hua Tseng: Schulz, T. J., et al. "Identification of inducible brown adipocyte progenitors residing in skeletal muscle and white fat." *Proc Natl Acad Sci USA* 108 (2011): 143–148.

A Japanese research team put subjects in an even milder setting: Saito, M., et al. "High incidence of metabolically active brown adipose tissue in healthy adult humans—effects of cold exposure and adiposity." *Diabetes* 58 (2009: 1526–1531.

In another study conducted by a group of Canadian researchers: Ouellet, V., et al. "Brown adipose tissue oxidative metabolism contributes to energy expenditure during acute cold exposure in humans." *J Clin Invest* 122 (2012): 545–552.

the herb bitter melon appears to increase activity of brown fat: Chan, L. L., et al. "Reduced adiposity in bitter melon (Momordica charantia)-fed rats is associated with increased lipid oxidative enzyme activities and uncoupling protein expression." *J Nutr* 135 (2005): 2517–2523.

ursolic acid—a substance that occurs in high concentrations in apple peels: Kunkel, S. D., et al. "Ursolic acid increases skeletal muscle and brown fat and decreases diet-induced obesity, glucose intolerance and fatty liver disease." *PLOS ONE* 7 (2012): e39332.

Studies have found that irisin, a newly identified hormone that is produced during exercise: Boström, P., et al. "A PGC1α-dependent myokine that drives browning of white fat and thermogenesis." *Nature* 481 (2012): 463–468.

Dr. Tseng and her colleagues published a study showing that BMP-7: Tseng, Y.-H, et al. "New role of bone morphogenetic protein 7 in brown adipogenesis and energy expenditure." *Nature* 454 (2008): 1000–1004.

STRATEGY CHAPTER 5

discovered that the molecule NF-KB, an important immune-system regulator found in fat and liver tissue: Cai, D., et al. "Local and systemic insulin resistance resulting from hepatic activation of IKK-β and NF-κB." *Nat Med* 11 (2005): 183–190.

in a 2001 study, they showed that aspirin can improve insulin sensitivity: Yuan, M., et al. "Reversal of obesity- and diet-induced insulin resistance with salicylates or targeted disruption of Ikkβ." *Science* 293 (2001): 1673–1677.

blood levels of C-reactive protein also correlate: Chou H. H., et al. "Insulin resistance is associated with C-reactive protein independent of abdominal obesity in nondiabetic Taiwanese." *Metabolism* 59 (2010): 824–830.

The Nurses Health Study, which followed 114,000 women for two decades: Hu, F. B., et al. "Diet, lifestyle, and the risk of type 2 diabetes mellitus in women." *N Engl J Med* 345 (2001): 790–797.

studies in the United Kingdom and Sweden have found that smokers: Nilsson, P. M., et al. "Smoking is associated with increased HbA1c values and microalbuminuria in patients with diabetes—data from the National Diabetes Register in Sweden." *Diabetes Metab* 30 (2004): 261–268.

CRP levels remain elevated in former cigarette smokers: Wannamethee, S. G., et al. "Associations between cigarette smoking, pipe/cigar smoking, and smoking cessation, and haemostatic and inflammatory markers for cardiovascular disease." *Eur Heart J* 26 (2005): 1765–1767.

at Columbia University, researchers reviewed twenty years' worth of data: Demmer, R. T., et al. "Periodontal disease and incident type 2 diabetes: results from the First National Health and Nutrition Examination Survey and its epidemiologic follow-up study." *Diabetes Care* 31 (2008): 1373–1379.

In a 2005 study, patients with well-controlled type 2 diabetes: Kiran, M., et al. "The effect of improved periodontal health on metabolic control in type 2 diabetes mellitus." *J Clin Periodontol* 32 (2005): 266–272.

Another study of individuals with type 2 diabetes and periodontal disease: Iwamoto, Y., et al. "The effect of antimicrobial periodontal treatment on circulating tumor necrosis factor alpha and glycated hemoglobin level in patients with type 2 diabetes." *J Periodontol* 72 (2001): 774–778.

In one recently published study, on which Joslin's Dr. Allison Goldfine: Pearson, J. F., et al. "Association between fine particulate matter and diabetes prevalence in the U.S." *Diabetes Care* 33 (2010): 2196–2201.

other research, including an animal study showing that exposure: Xu, X., et al. "Effect of early particulate air pollution exposure on obesity in mice: role of p47phox." *Arterioscler Thromb Vasc Biol* 30 (2010): 2518–2527.

Mayo Clinic researchers found that the risk of developing type 2 diabetes was doubled: Yun, H. D., et al. "Asthma and proinflammatory conditions: a population-based retrospective matched cohort study." *Mayo Clin Proc* 87 (2012): 953–960.

curcumin supplements can reduce inflammation-related symptoms: Chandran, B., et al. "A randomized, pilot study to assess the efficacy and safety of curcumin in patients with active rheumatoid arthritis." *Phytother Res* 26 (2012): 1719–1725.

In a randomized clinical trial conducted at Joslin several years ago: Goldfine, A. B., et al. "The effects of salsalate on glycemic control in patients with type 2 diabetes: a randomized trial." *Ann Intern Med* 152 (2010): 346–357.

researchers published the Stage 2 results of the clinical trial: Goldfine, A. B., et al. "Salicylate (salsalate) in patients with type 2 diabetes: a randomized trial." *Ann Intern Med* 159 (2013): 1–12.

the University of Pennsylvania compared 108,132 people with psoriasis: Azfar, R. S., et al. "Increased risk of diabetes and likelihood of receiving diabetes treatment in patients with psoriasis." *Arch Dermatol* 148 (2012): 995–1000.

A recent analysis of population data by researchers at Brigham and Women's Hospital: Solomon, D. H., et al. "Risk of diabetes among patients with rheumatoid arthritis, psoriatic arthritis and psoriasis." *Ann Rheum Dis* 69 (2010): 2114–2117.

STRATEGY CHAPTER 6

first study attempting to simulate a more realistic "lack of sleep" scenario: Spiegel, K., et al. "Impact of sleep debt on metabolic and endocrine function." *Lancet* (354) 1999: 1435–1439.

A 2011 analysis by the Centers for Disease Control and Prevention: Centers for Disease Control and Prevention. "Unhealthy Sleep-Related Behaviors—12 States, 2009." *MMWR* 60 (2011): 233–238.

between 50 and 70 million Americans have chronic sleep disorders: Institute of Medicine. "Sleep disorders and sleep deprivation: an unmet public health problem." The National Academies Press (2006).

Americans get one and a half to two hours less sleep per night: National Sleep Foundation. "Sleep in America" poll. National Sleep Foundation (2002).

Another important University of Chicago study, published in 2009: Nedeltcheva, A.V., et al. "Exposure to recurrent sleep restriction in the setting of high caloric intake and physical inactivity results in increased insulin resistance and reduced glucose tolerance." *J Clin Endocrinol Metab* 94 (2009): 3242–3250.

An even more recent study at Leiden University Medical Center: Donga, E., et al. "A single night of partial sleep deprivation induces insulin resistance in multiple metabolic pathways in healthy subjects." *J Clin Endocrinol Metab* 95 (2010): 2963–2968.

Especially convincing was a recent University of Chicago study: Broussard, J. L., et al. "Impaired insulin signaling in human adipocytes after experimental sleep restriction: a randomized, crossover study." *Ann Intern Med* 157 (2012): 549–557.

An analysis of a cross-section of nearly 1,500 men and women: Gottlieb, D. J., et al. "Association of sleep time with diabetes mellitus and impaired glucose tolerance." *Arch Intern Med* 165 (2005): 863–867.

the Massachusetts Male Aging Study, which followed 1,700 men: Yaggi, H. K., et al. "Sleep duration as a risk factor for the development of type 2 diabetes." *Diabetes Care* 29 (2006): 657–661.

published in 2010 by researchers at the University of Warwick: Cappuccio, F. P., et al. "Quantity and quality of sleep and incidence of type 2 diabetes: a systematic review and meta-analysis." *Diabetes Care* 33 (2010): 414–420.

A U.S. study published in 2010 that analyzed data from nearly 1,500 subjects: Rafalson, L., et al. "Short sleep duration is associated with the development of impaired fasting glucose: The Western New York Health Study." *Ann Epidemiol* 20 (2010): 883–889.

One of the largest such studies, the Sleep Heart Health Study: Punjabi, N. M., et al. "Sleep-disordered breathing, glucose intolerance, and insulin resistance: the Sleep Heart Health Study." *Am J Epidemiol* 160 (2004): 521–530.

the University of Chicago evaluated sixty subjects with type 2 diabetes: Aronsohn, R. S., et al. "Impact of untreated obstructive sleep apnea on glucose control in type 2 diabetes." *Am J Respir Crit Care Med* 181 (2010): 507–513.

Another Swedish study followed more than 2,600 middle-aged men: Elmasry A., et al. "The role of habitual snoring and obesity in the development of diabetes: A 10-year follow-up study in a male population." *J Intern Med* 248 (2000): 13–20.

An analysis of 70,000 women who participated in the Nurses' Health Study: Al-Delaimy W. K., et al. "Snoring as a risk factor for type II diabetes mellitus: a prospective study." *Am J Epidemiol* 155 (2002): 387–393.

Yale researchers published results of a six-year study involving nearly six hundred non-diabetic people: Botros, N., et al. "Obstructive sleep apnea as a risk factor for type 2 diabetes." *Am J Med* 122 (2009): 1122–1127.

In the NEJM study, most of the 126 patients it followed: Strollo, P. J. Jr., et al. "Upper-airway stimulation for obstructive sleep apnea." *N Engl J Med* 370 (2014): 139–149.

STRATEGY CHAPTER 7

Israeli researchers concluded that exposure to a single intense episode: Boaz, M., et al. "Institutional point-of-care glucometer identifies population trends in blood glucose associated with war." *Diabetes Technol Ther* 15 (2013): 964–967.

In a Dutch study published in 2000, researchers gave more than 2,200 subjects: Mooy, J. M., et al. "Major stressful life events in relation to prevalence of undetected type 2 diabetes." *Diabetes Care* 23 (2000): 197–201.

Another study, published in 2004, looked at data on nearly six thousand people: Goodwin, R. D., et al. "Association between childhood trauma and physical disorders among adults in the United States." *Psychol Med* 34 (2004): 509–520.

Finnish and U.S. researchers identified more than five hundred middle-aged women: Räikkönen, K., et al. "Depressive symptoms and stressful life events predict metabolic syndrome among middle-aged women: a comparison of World Health Organization, Adult Treatment Panel III, and International Diabetes Foundation definitions." *Diabetes Care* 30 (2007): 872–877.

Even more striking, a Japanese study: Kato, M., et al. "Psychological factors, coffee and risk of diabetes mellitus among middle-aged Japanese: a population-based prospective study in the JPHC study cohort." *Endocr J* 56 (2009): 459–468.

Another Japanese study, published in 2008: Toshihiro, M., et al. "Psychosocial factors are independent risk factors for the development of Type 2 diabetes in Japanese workers with impaired fasting glucose and/or impaired glucose tolerance." *Diabet Med* 25 (2008): 1211–1217.

Native Hawaiians who lived a traditional lifestyle: Kaholokula, J. K., et al. "Association between acculturation modes and type 2 diabetes among Native Hawaiians." *Diabetes Care* 31 (2008): 698–700.

published by a research team from the Netherlands in 2006: Knol, M. J., et al. "Depression as a risk factor for the onset of type 2 diabetes mellitus. A meta-analysis." *Diabetologia* 49 (2006): 837–845.

researchers at Johns Hopkins University and the University of Michigan: Mezuk, B., et al. "Depression and type 2 diabetes over the lifespan: a meta-analysis." *Diabetes Care* 31 (2008): 2383–2390.

A large Norwegian study of 37,000 men and women: Engum, A. "The role of depression and anxiety in onset of diabetes in a large population-based study." *J Psychosom Res* 62 (2007): 31–38.

a meta-analysis of sixteen human studies, published in 2008: Blaine, B. "Does depression cause obesity?: A meta-analysis of longitudinal studies of depression and weight control." *J Health Psychol* 13 (2008): 1190–1197.

a prospective study that followed more than ten thousand British civil servants: Chandola, T., et al. "Chronic stress at work and the metabolic syndrome: prospective study." *BMJ* 332 (2006): 521–525.

a recent Swedish study that followed 5,400 women and men: Eriksson, A. K., et al. "Work stress, sense of coherence, and risk of type 2 diabetes in a prospective study of middle-aged Swedish men and women." *Diabetes Care* 36 (2013): 2683–2689.

a research study that followed 4,300 middle-aged British civil servants: Kivimäki, M., et al. "Common mental disorder and obesity: insight from four repeat measures over 19 years: prospective Whitehall II cohort study." *BMJ* 339 (2009): b3765.

A meta-analysis of eleven studies: Roshanaei-Moghaddam, B., et al. "The longitudinal effects of depression on physical activity." *Gen Hosp Psychiatry* 31 (2009): 306–315.

data from the Coronary Artery Risk Development in Young Adults Study: Needham, B. L., et al. "Trajectories of change in obesity and symptoms of depression: the CARDIA study." *Am J Public Health* 100 (2010): 1040–1046.

a 1998 British study of 370 men ages sixty to seventy: Phillips, D. I., et al. "Elevated plasma cortisol concentrations: a link between low birth weight and the insulin resistance syndrome?" *J Clin Endocrinol Metab* 83 (1998): 757–760.

twelve sessions of CBT not only improved symptoms: Levy-Gigi, E., et al. "Association among clinical response, hippocampal volume, and FKBP5 gene expression in individuals with posttraumatic stress disorder receiving cognitive behavioral therapy." *Biol Psychiatry* 74 (2013): 793–800.

a review of multiple meta-analyses published in 2010 concluded that CBT: Olatunji, B. O., et al. "Efficacy of cognitive behavioral therapy for anxiety disorders: a review of meta-analytic findings." *Psychiatr Clin North Am* 33 (2010): 557–577.

A 2010 review paper looked at eight different meta-analyses: Shedler, J. "The efficacy of psychodynamic psychotherapy." *Am Psychol* 65 (2010): 98–109.

STRATEGY CHAPTER 8

a recent study coauthored by Dr. C. Ronald Kahn: Ristow, M., et al. "Antioxidants prevent health-promoting effects of physical exercise in humans." *Proc Natl Acad Sci USA* 106 (2009): 8665–8670.

A 2011 meta-analysis of the glucose-control effects of vitamin E: Suksomboon, N., et al. "Effects of vitamin E supplementation on glycaemic control in type 2 diabetes: systematic review of randomized controlled trials." *J Clin Pharm Ther* 36 (2011): 53–63.

A 2008 analysis of data from a large-scale prospective European study: Harding, A. H., et al. "Plasma vitamin C level, fruit and vegetable consumption, and the risk of new-onset type 2 diabetes mellitus: the European prospective investigation of cancer–Norfolk prospective study." *Arch Intern Med* 168 (2008): 1493–1499.

In one recent meta-analysis of twenty-one studies involving more than 76,000 individuals: Song, Y., et al. "Blood 25-hydroxy vitamin D levels and incident type 2 diabetes: a meta-analysis of prospective studies." *Diabetes Care* 36 (2013): 1422–1428.

In 2011, investigators at the NIH's National Institute for Aging: Beydoun, M. A., et al. "Serum antioxidant status is associated with metabolic syndrome among U.S. adults in recent national surveys." *J Nutr* 141 (2011): 903–913.

an analysis of nearly eight hundred American adolescents: Beydoun, M. A., et al. "Serum antioxidant concentrations and metabolic syndrome are associated among U.S. adolescents in recent national surveys." *J Nutr* 142 (2012): 1693–1704.

Greek researchers looked at a subset of more than one thousand men and women: Psaltopoulou, T., et al. "Dietary antioxidant capacity is inversely associated with diabetes biomarkers: the ATTICA study." *Nutr Metab Cardiovasc Dis* 21 (2011): 561–567.

In a 2006 paper published in the journal **Nature:** Houstis, N., et al. "Reactive oxygen species have a causal role in multiple forms of insulin resistance." *Nature* 440 (2006): 944–948.

Investigators in France have found fascinating evidence that impaired mitochondrial function: Bonnard, C., et al. "Mitochondrial dysfunction results from oxidative stress in the skeletal muscle of diet-induced insulin-resistant mice." *J Clin Invest* 118 (2008): 789–800.

STRATEGIES TO PREVENT OR CONTROL GESTATIONAL DIABETES

a ground-breaking 2012 study by researchers at the National Institutes of Health: Bowers, K., et al. "A prospective study of prepregnancy dietary fat intake and risk of gestational diabetes." *Am J Clin Nutr* 95 (2012): 446–453.

A meta-analysis led by Harvard researchers found that the women who were most active: Tobias, D. K., et al. "Physical activity before and during pregnancy and risk of gestational diabetes mellitus: a meta-analysis." *Diabetes Care* 34 (2011): 223–229.

A recently published NIH study analyzed data compiled by the Nurses' Health Study II: Bao, W., et al. "Physical activity and sedentary behaviors associated with risk of progression from gestational diabetes mellitus to type 2 diabetes mellitus: a prospective cohort study." *JAMA Intern Med* 174 (2014): 1047–1055.

INDEX